Dedicated to my children and others who exemplify hope and healing,
inspiring those around them never to underestimate
the power of a healthy lifestyle.

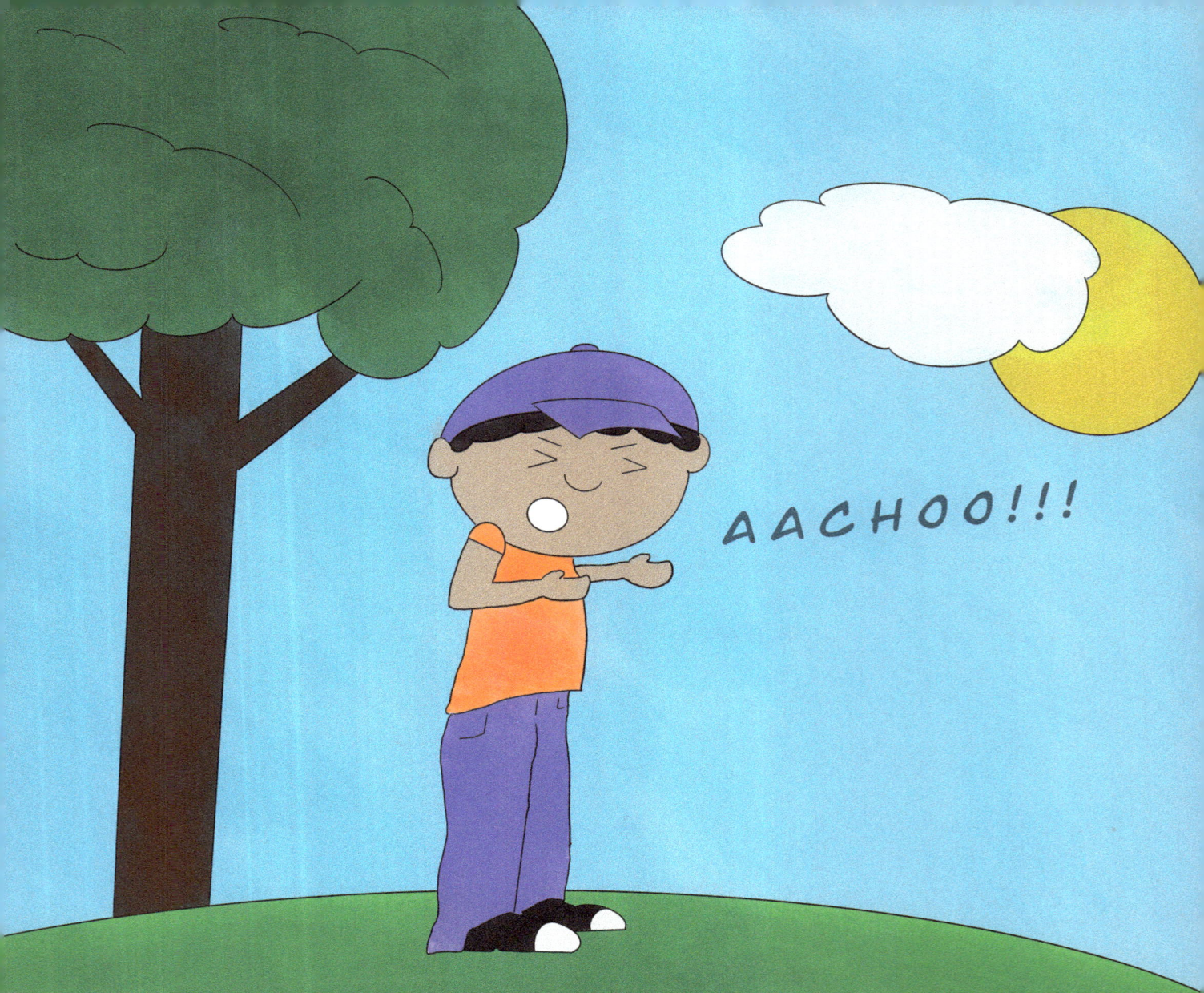

"Aachoo!" Adam sneezes, running through the yard, he immediately stops as he holds his chest. "Why can't I run like the other kids?" He thought.

Adam scurries back inside the house. "Mom, how come every time I run, my body stops me, I can't breathe and I sneeze?"

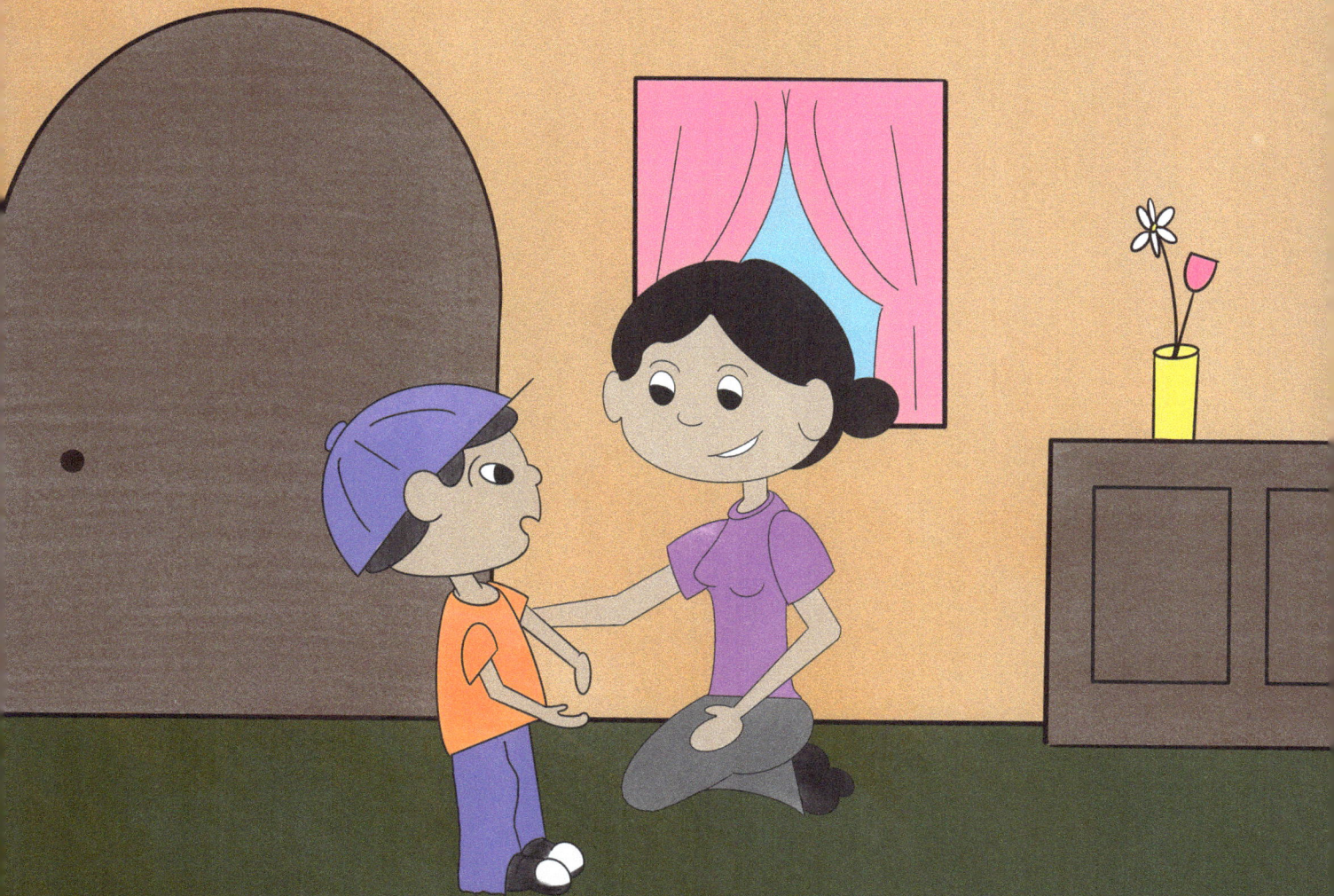

Mom picks Adam up and puts him on her lap, "Your body is different than other kids, you have asthma and allergies. See this rash on your body, you also have eczema, but that's what makes you super special. Now clean up, it is time to go meet all your friends at the picnic."

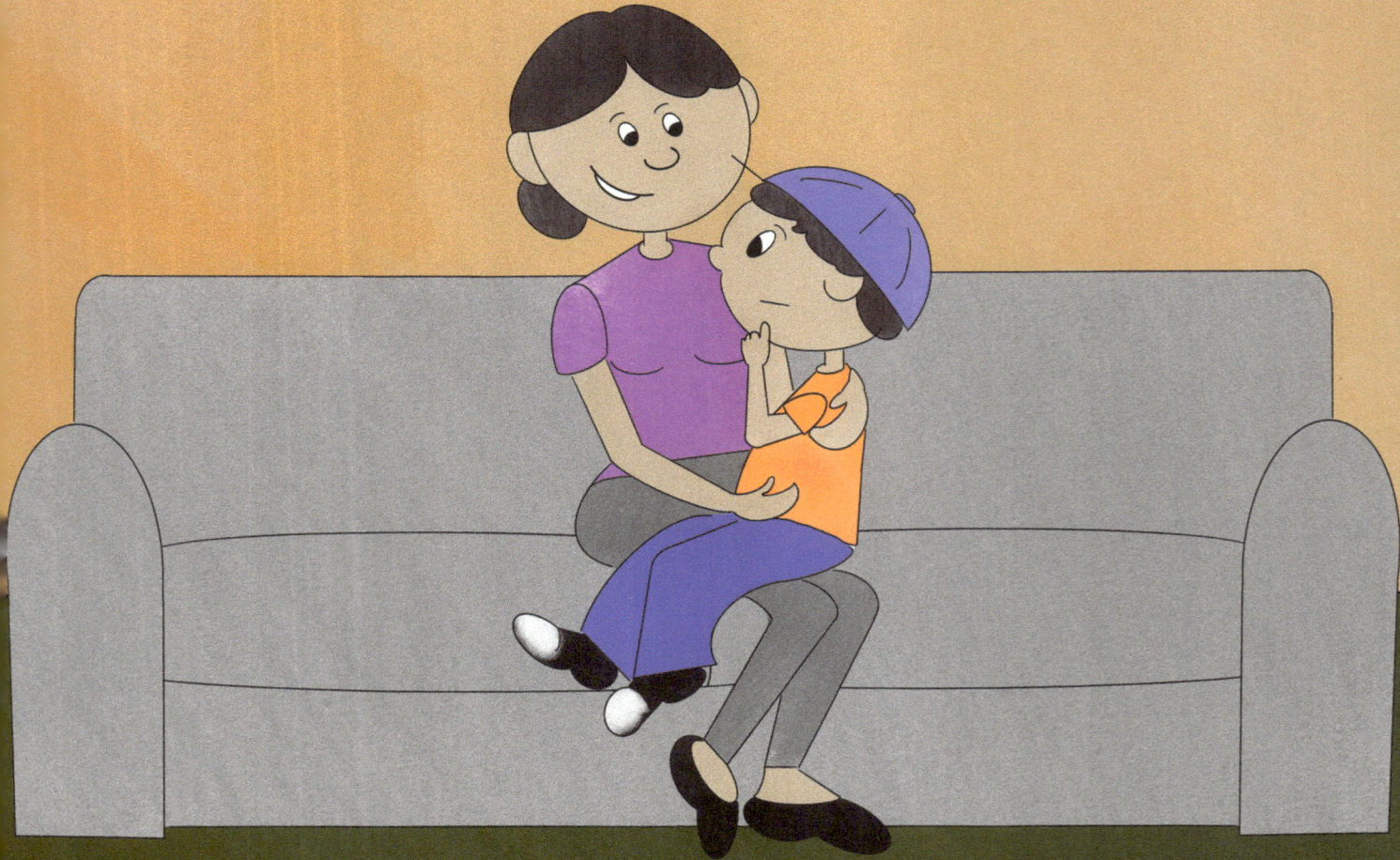

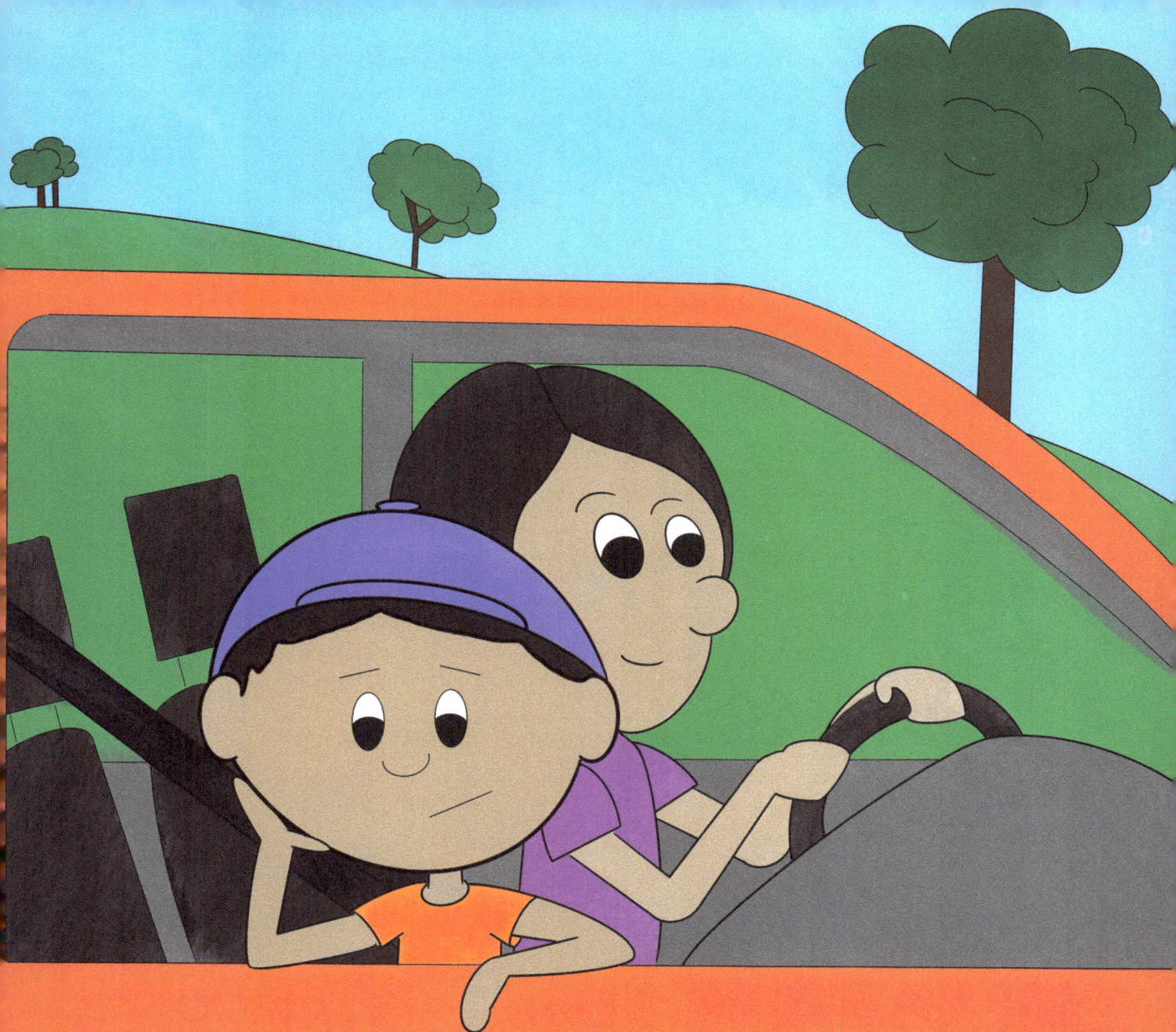

On the way to the picnic, Adam wondered, why do I have asthma, why do I have allergies, why do I have eczema, and my friends don't?

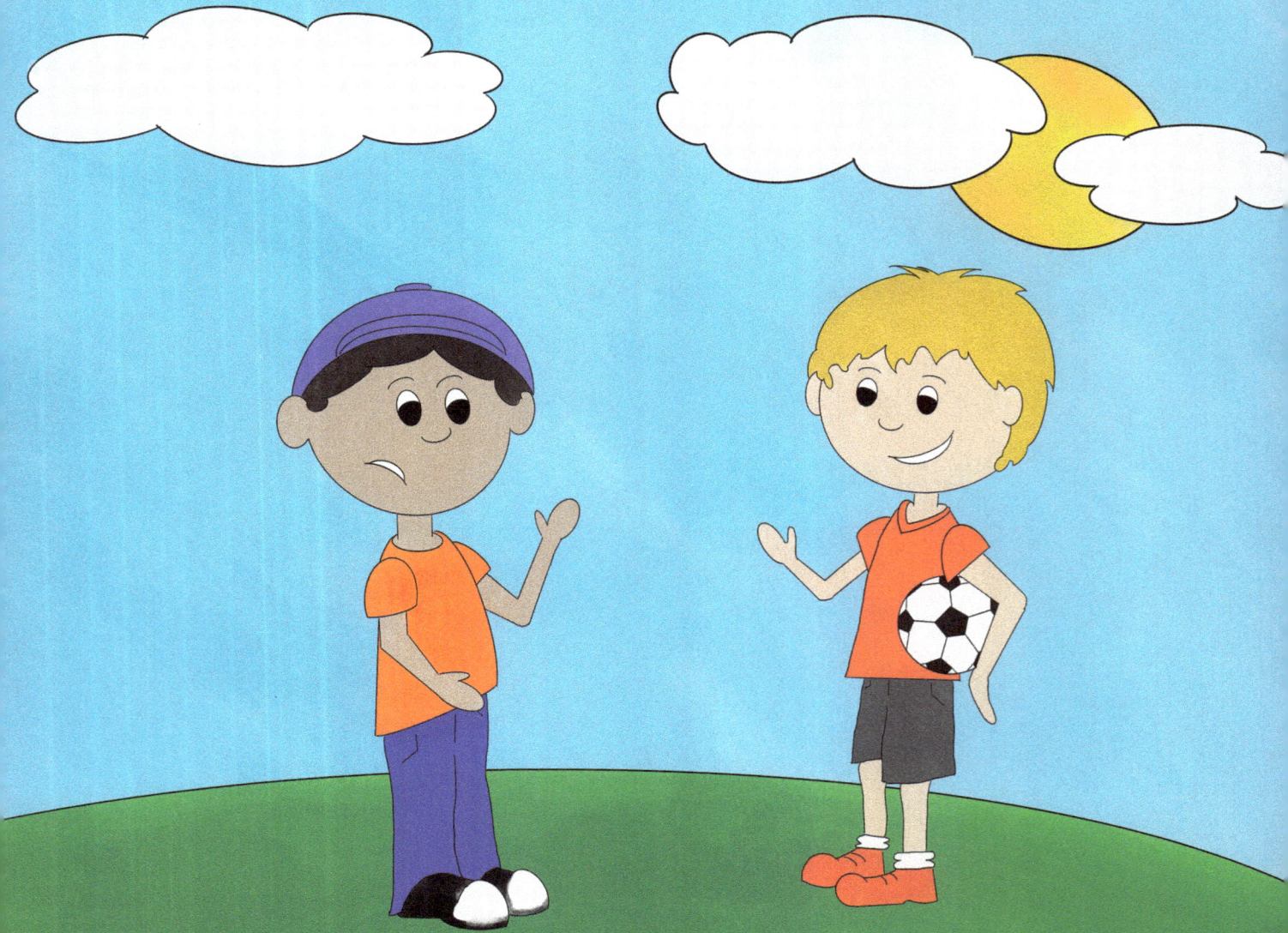

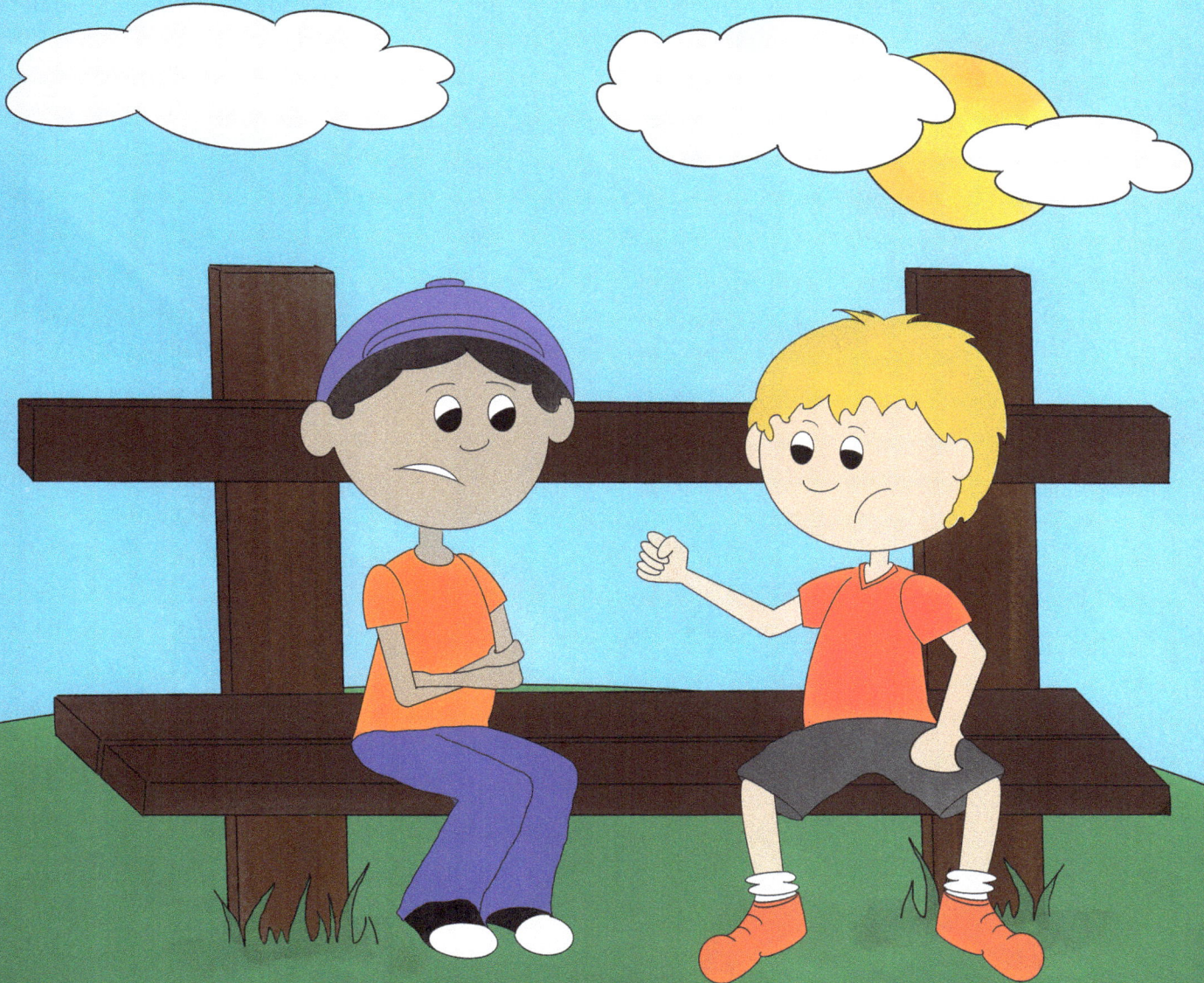
Noah sits next to his friend. "Did you know I also had eczema? My arm itched, it burned and I felt so tired all the time, I was just like you."

Adam's eyes widened in curiosity, "Really? But where is the rash now?"
Noah told him that it was gone when his mommy took him to a holistic doctor.

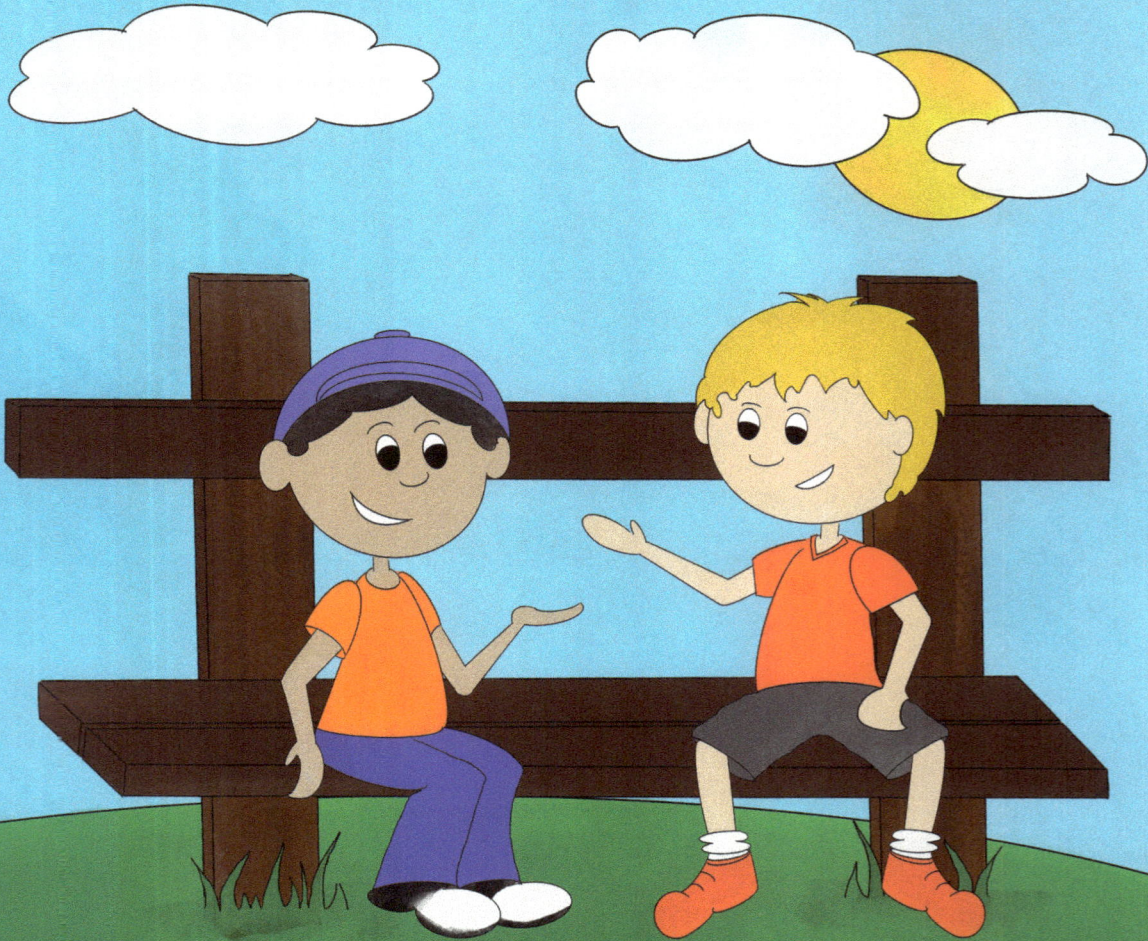

The holistic doctor looks at the whole body, not just parts of the body,
to figure out why there is a problem.

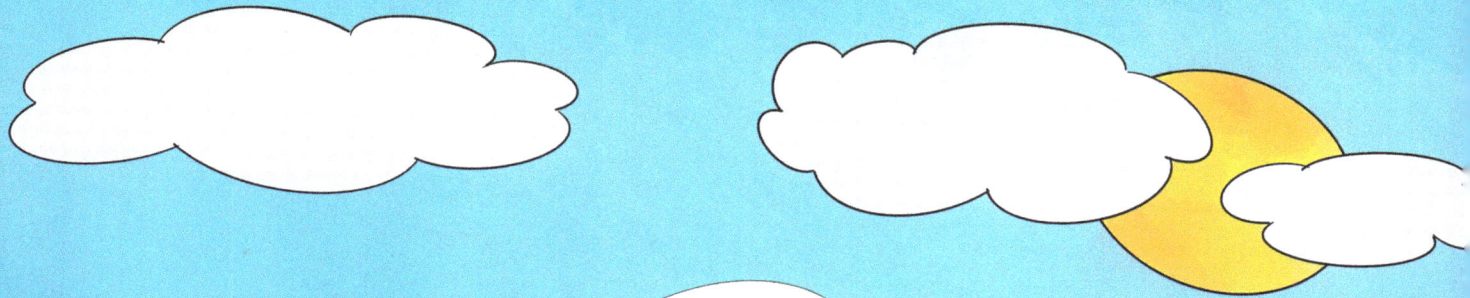

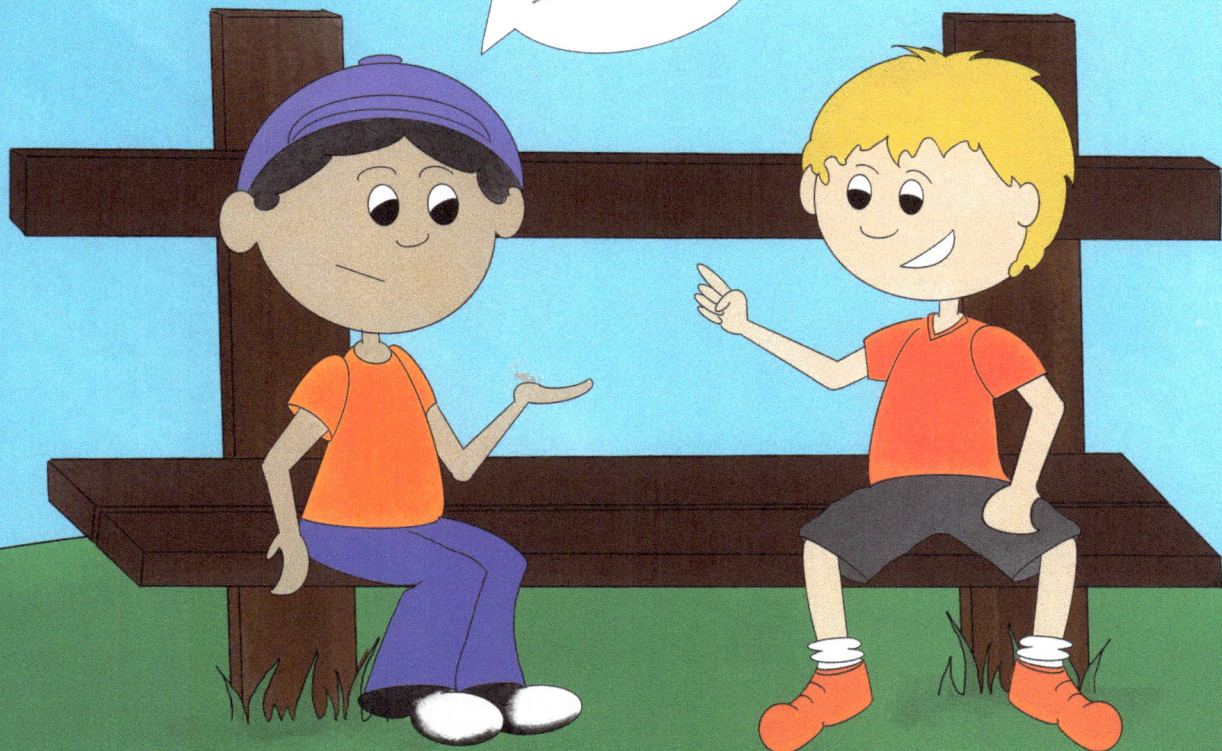

Noah reassures Adam, "No, not that type of fire, this is created by our immune cells and helps us feel better. But when the fire stays on for too long, it can turn to bad fire—that makes us very sick."

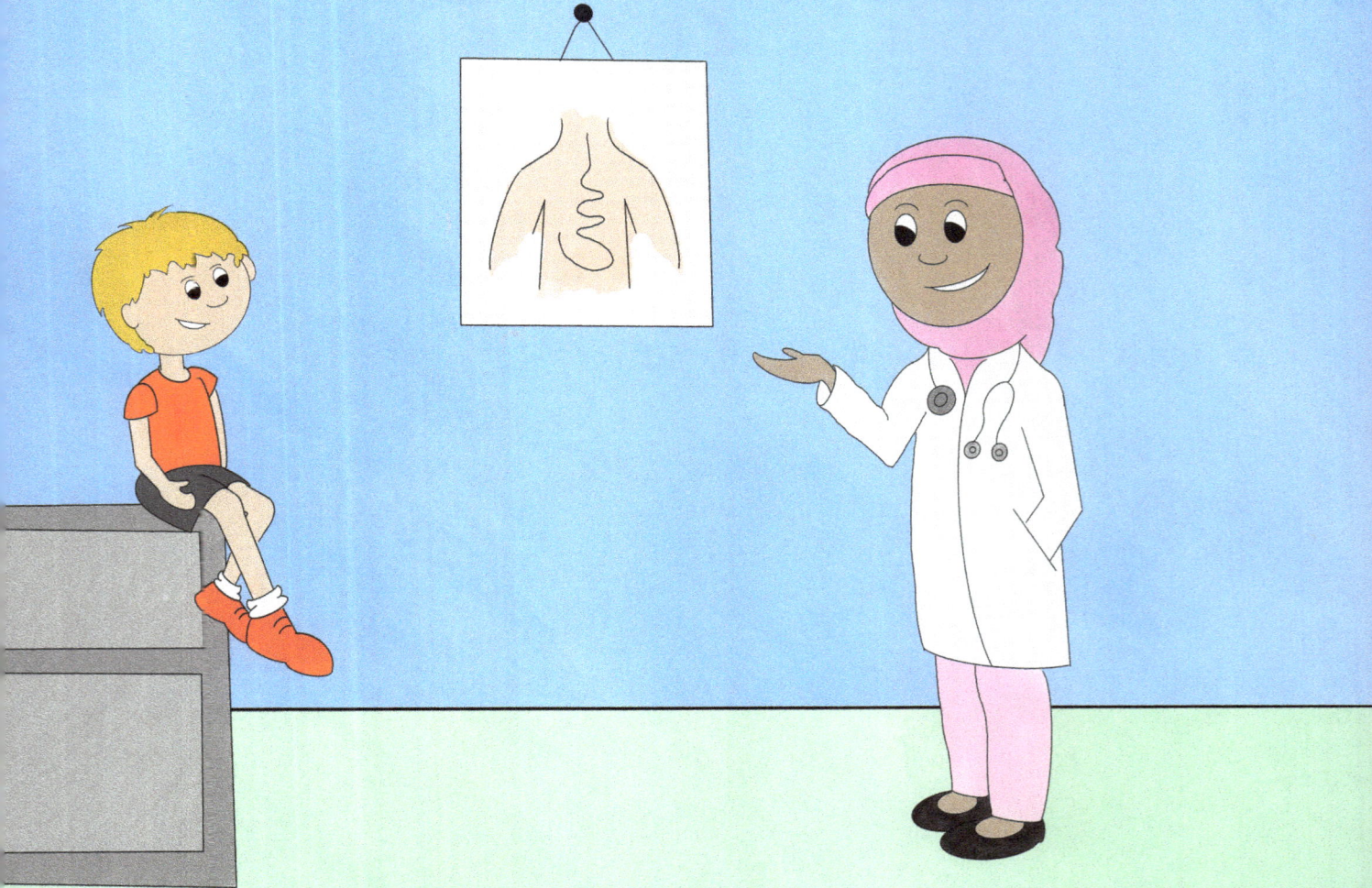

The doctor taught my mom and me how to protect our blessings—our bodies and our health. It took time, but now I don't have eczema anymore and can run like all the other kids.

Adam's frown turned upside down. When we take care of our body, we help everything work better, put out this bad fire and help our body heal itself.

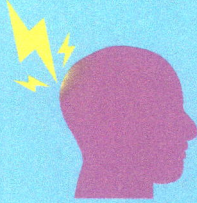

STRESS MANAGEMENT

HAPPY GUT

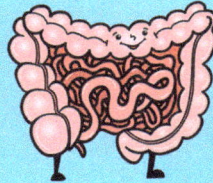

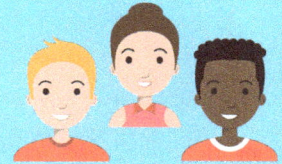

PLAY WITH GOOD FRIENDS

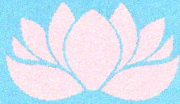

GRATITUDE

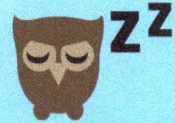

SLEEP

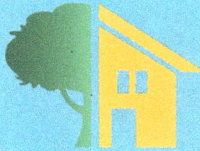

CLEAN ENVIRONMENT

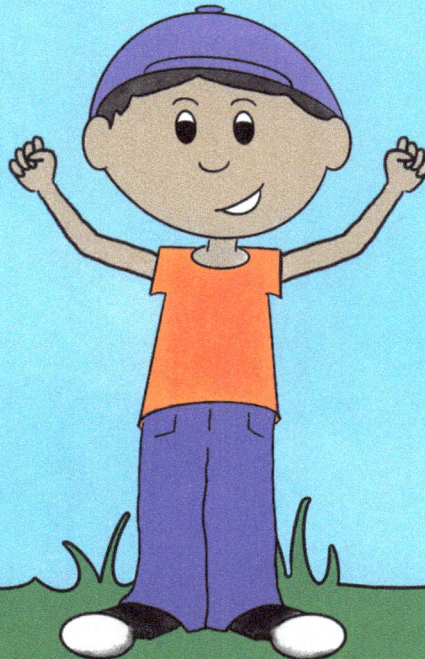

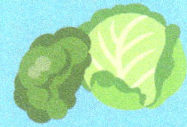

REAL FOOD & DRINK

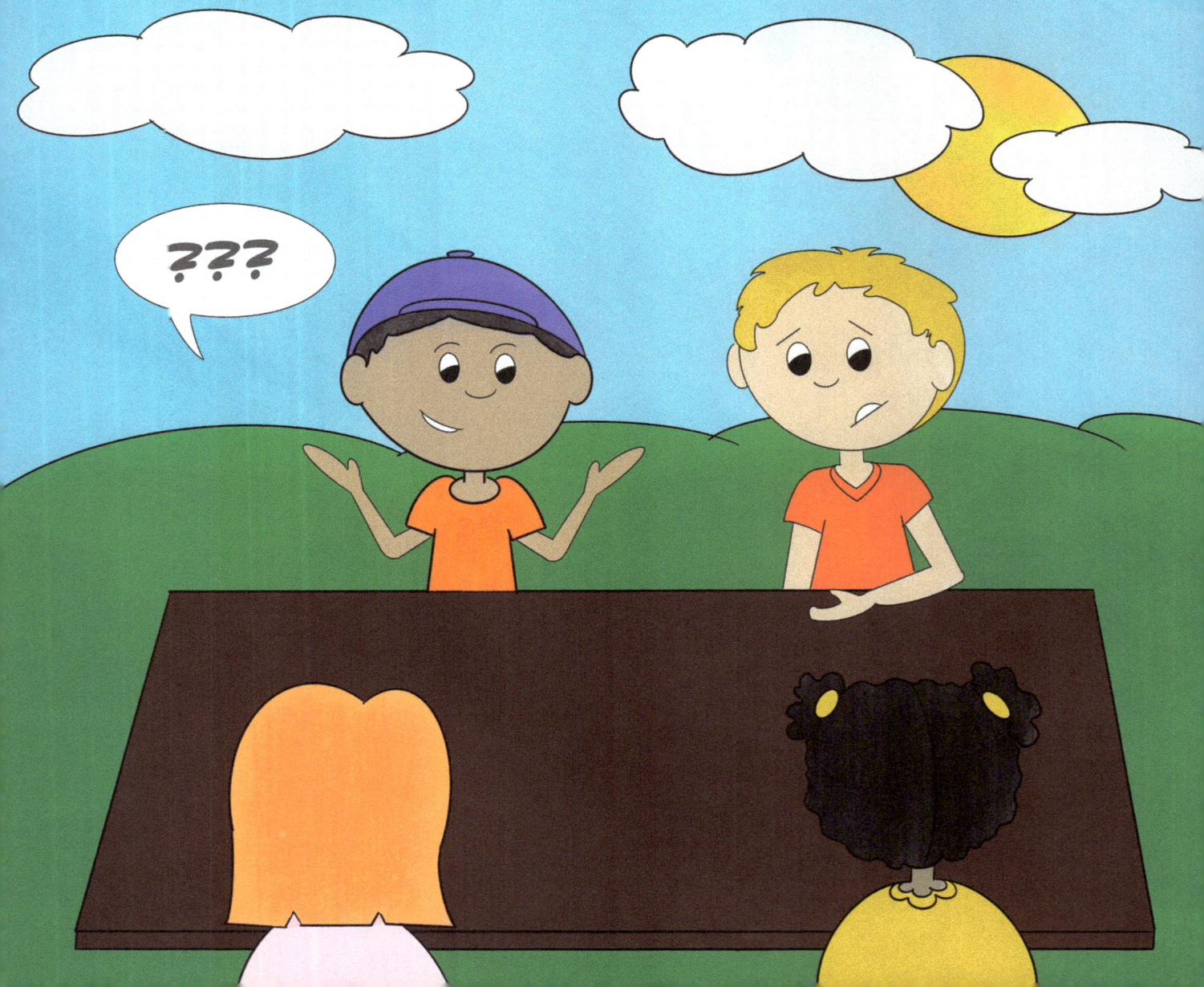

Mary and Sophia see their friends at the picnic table.
They run over to join Adam and Noah. Adam asks,
"What do you guys do to take care of your bodies?"

Noah starts, "I wake up every morning, and mommy and I sing the thankful song. Mom starts by singing, 'Thank you for my ears, thank you for my eyes, thank you for another beautiful day!'

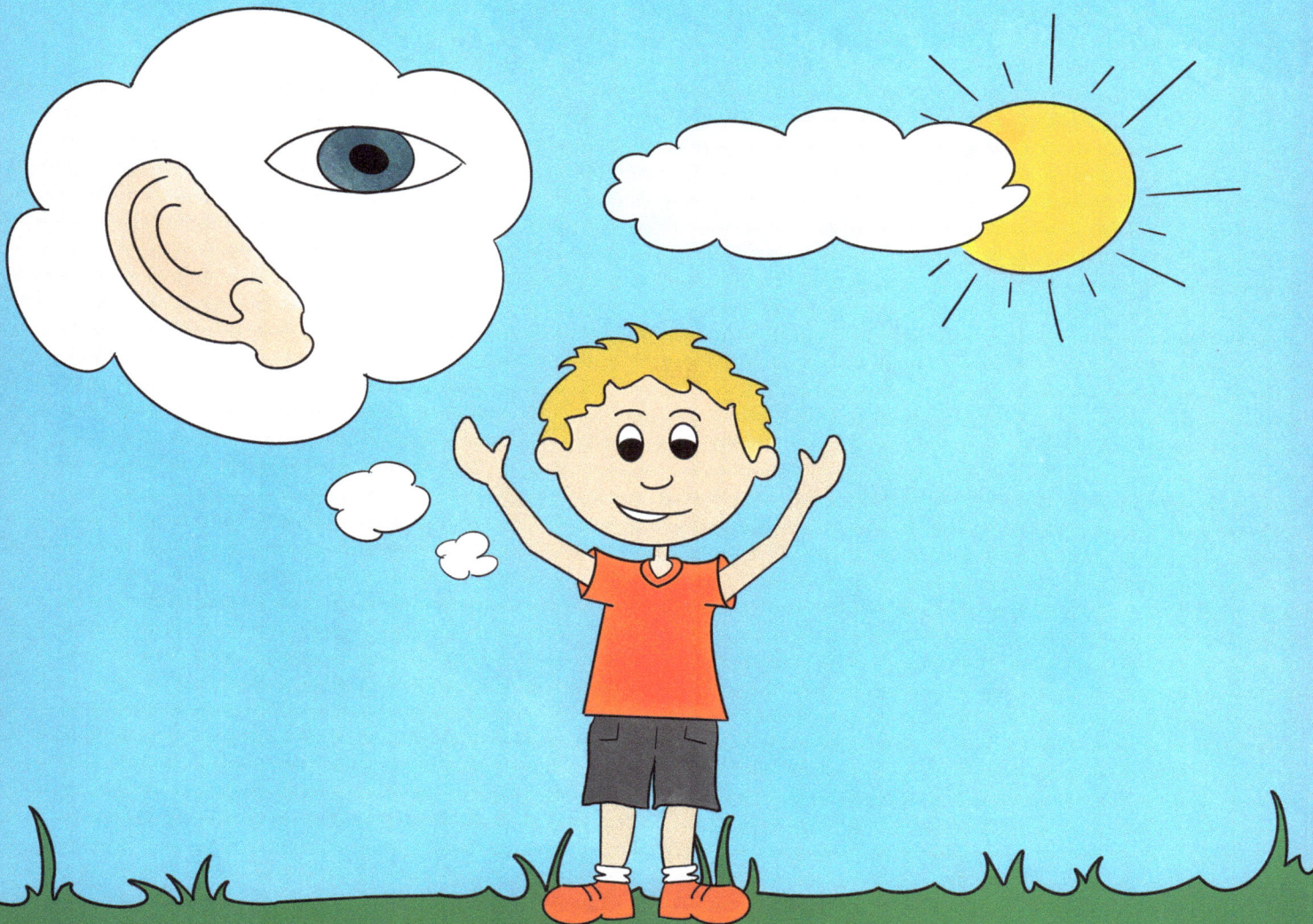

Then we take turns! It is so much fun, especially when my little brother starts saying he's thankful for his belly button!" Noah laughed.
"My mom says we should concentrate on what is good in our lives and all our blessings, instead of what is bad in our lives and what we don't have."

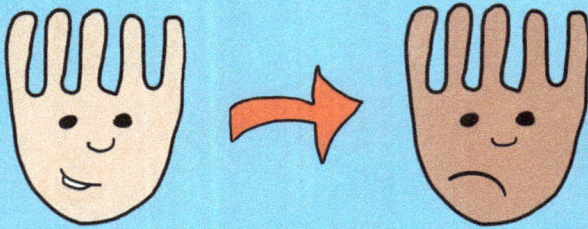

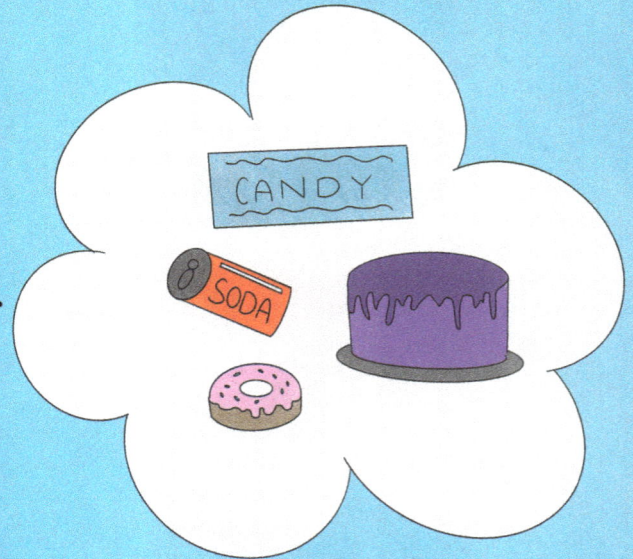

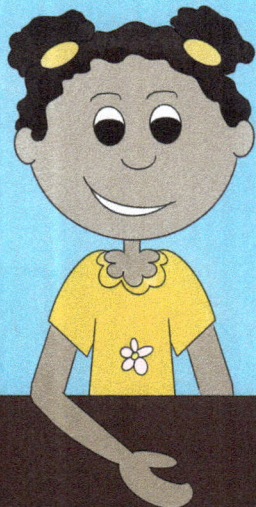

Noah jumps in. "Remember to drink lots of water! We have lots of soup made with bone broth that keeps my tummy healthy.

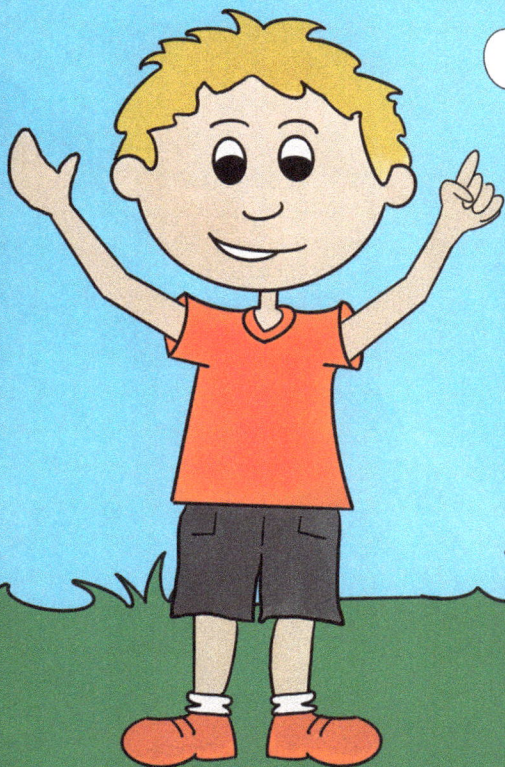

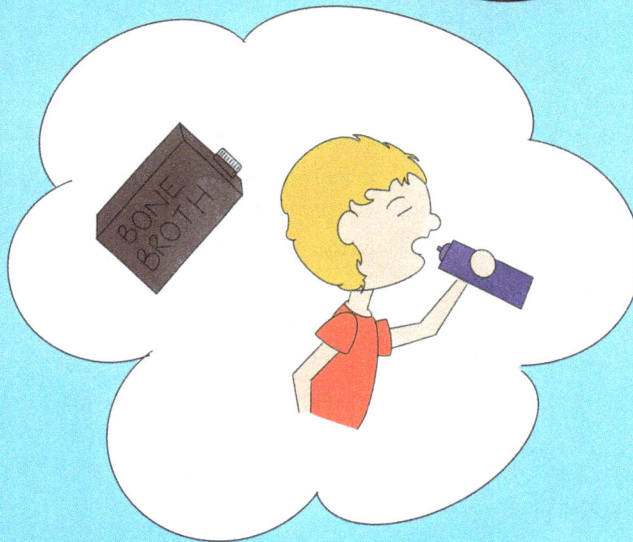

Other things I love are when my mom makes a green hulk smoothie, and I drink lots of filtered water! So refreshing! I love lemon water first thing in the morning!"

Mary adds, "Our little friends love the rainbow. We need lots of veggies, protein, like salmon, and healthy fat like avocado, nuts, and olives and oooh all the colorful fruit! So, whenever I am hungry, I always go down the list...

Veggies
Protein
Healthy Fat
Fruit

I LOVE EATING THE RAINBOW!

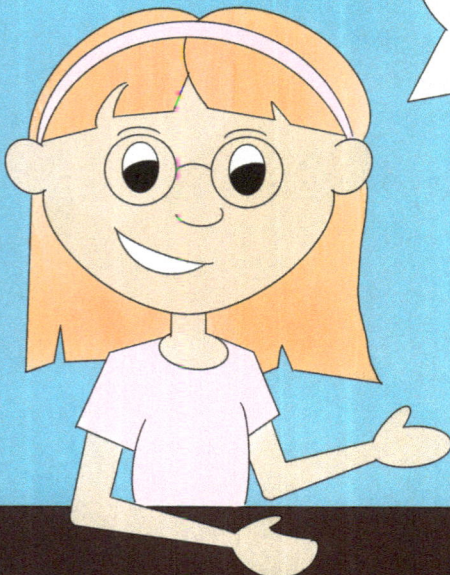

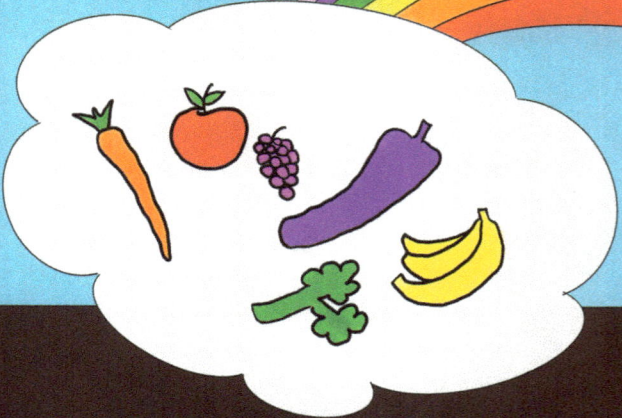

to make sure I have all the foods my lil' friends need to be strong. I love eating the rainbow...it makes me so happy!"

"If I eat rice or other grains, it usually fills me up and then I don't eat a lot of veggies. So, my mom always gives me lots of veggies first because my lil' friends and my body need veggies to stay fit. My favorites are broccoli, mushrooms, and cabbage, like sauerkraut! My lil' friends in my belly love sauerkraut!

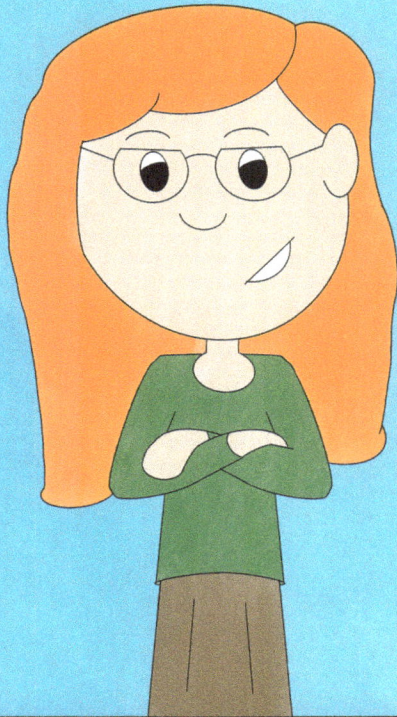

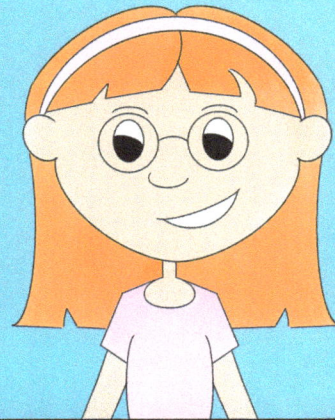

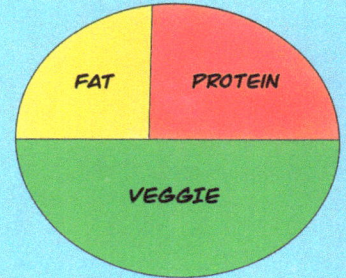

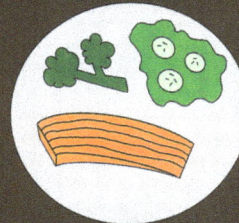

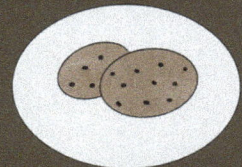

FAT
PROTEIN
VEGGIE

Mmm... if I want waffles, cookies or cake, my mom will make them out of almond or coconut flour. It's sooo delicious and keeps me full for a long time!" They all start cheering, "We love cookies!"

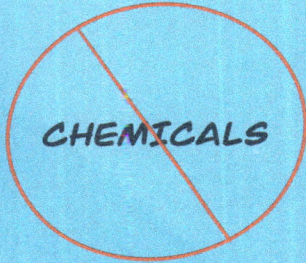

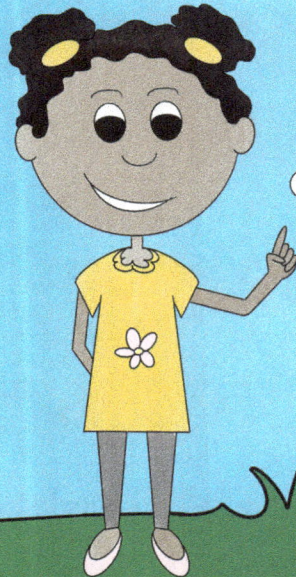

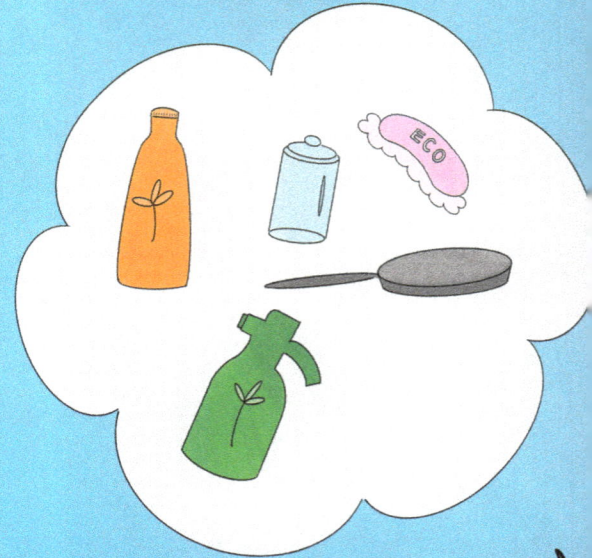

"We wash our clothes with natural laundry soap, clean the house with sprays all without chemicals. Mom even uses cast iron or glass to cook with and store stuff in. By doing this, it keeps chemicals far, far away from me and my friends. My lil' friends hate chemicals."

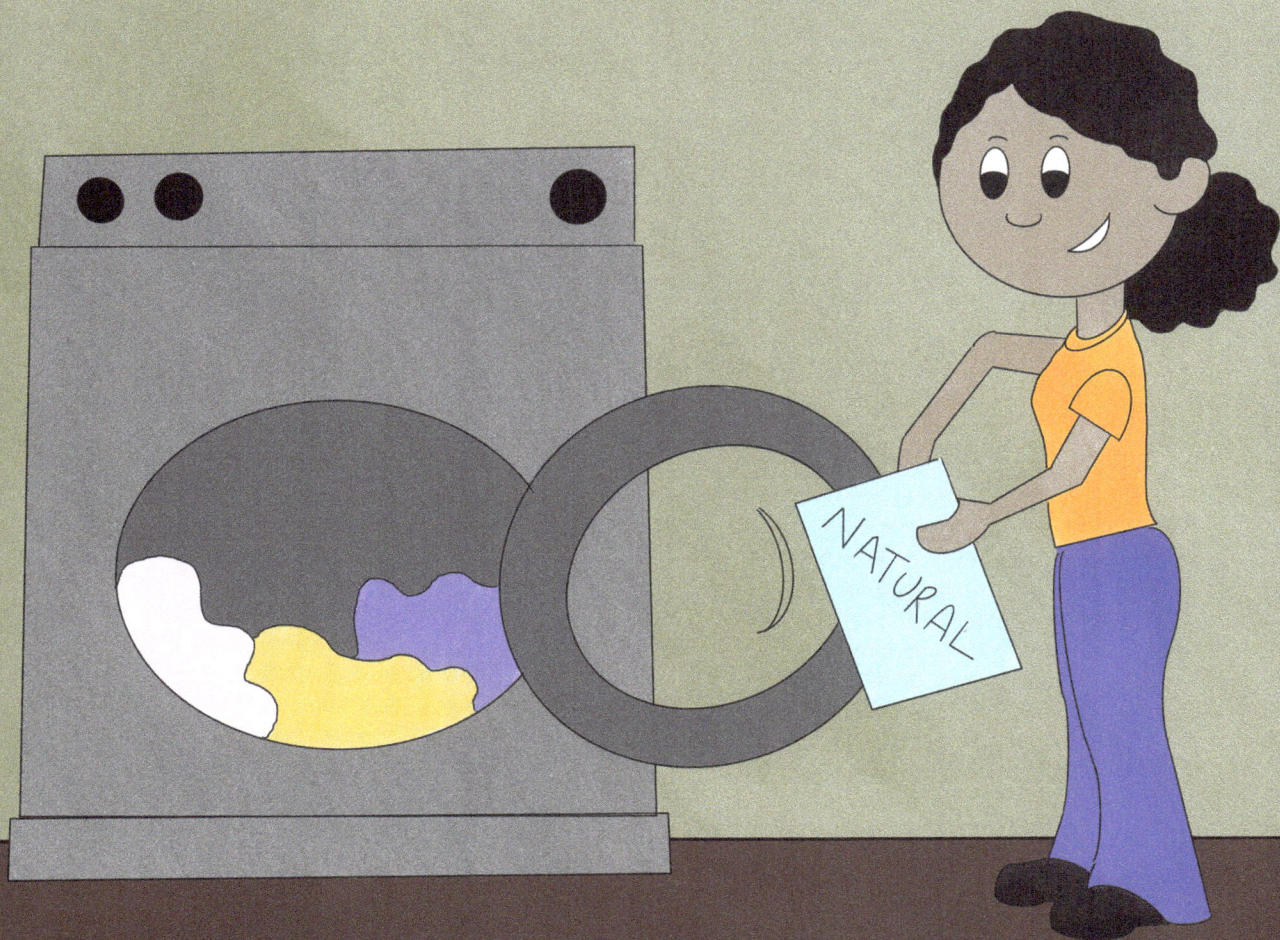

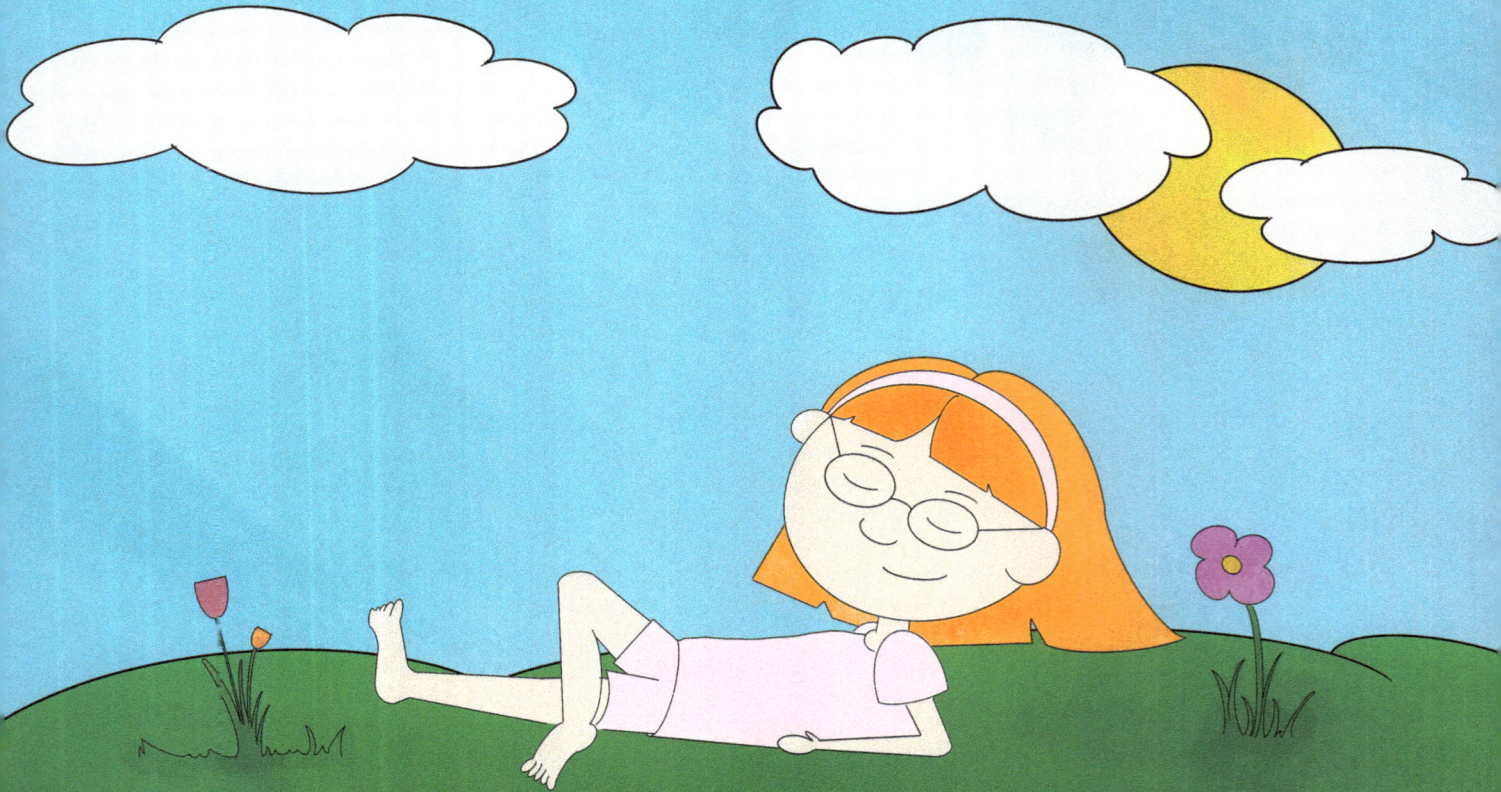

Mary claims, "Ooo and I love to play outside! Did you know being with friends and playing outside can keep you healthy and happy?"

Playing outside in the grass, sometimes without shoes, is my favorite and it can also help our immune system by adding more lil' friends in our bodies.

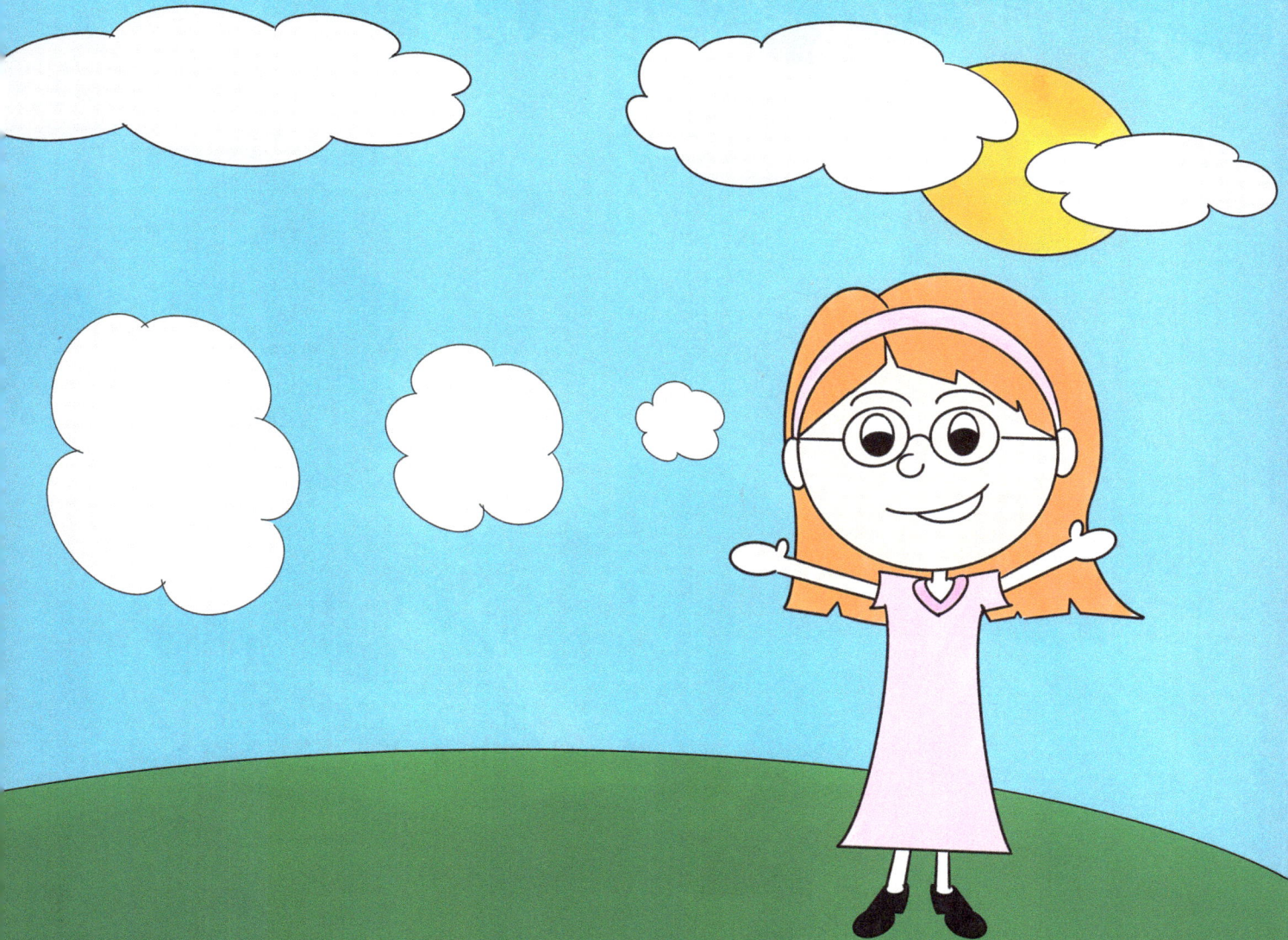

The more different kinds of good friends
in our bellies the better our health! Yay!

Noah continues, "After dinner, I have a bedtime routine. I play with my family and then one hour before I go to bed, we clean the house and then practice our breathing techniques, meditation and focus on what we are feeling at that moment, that is called *mindfulness*—

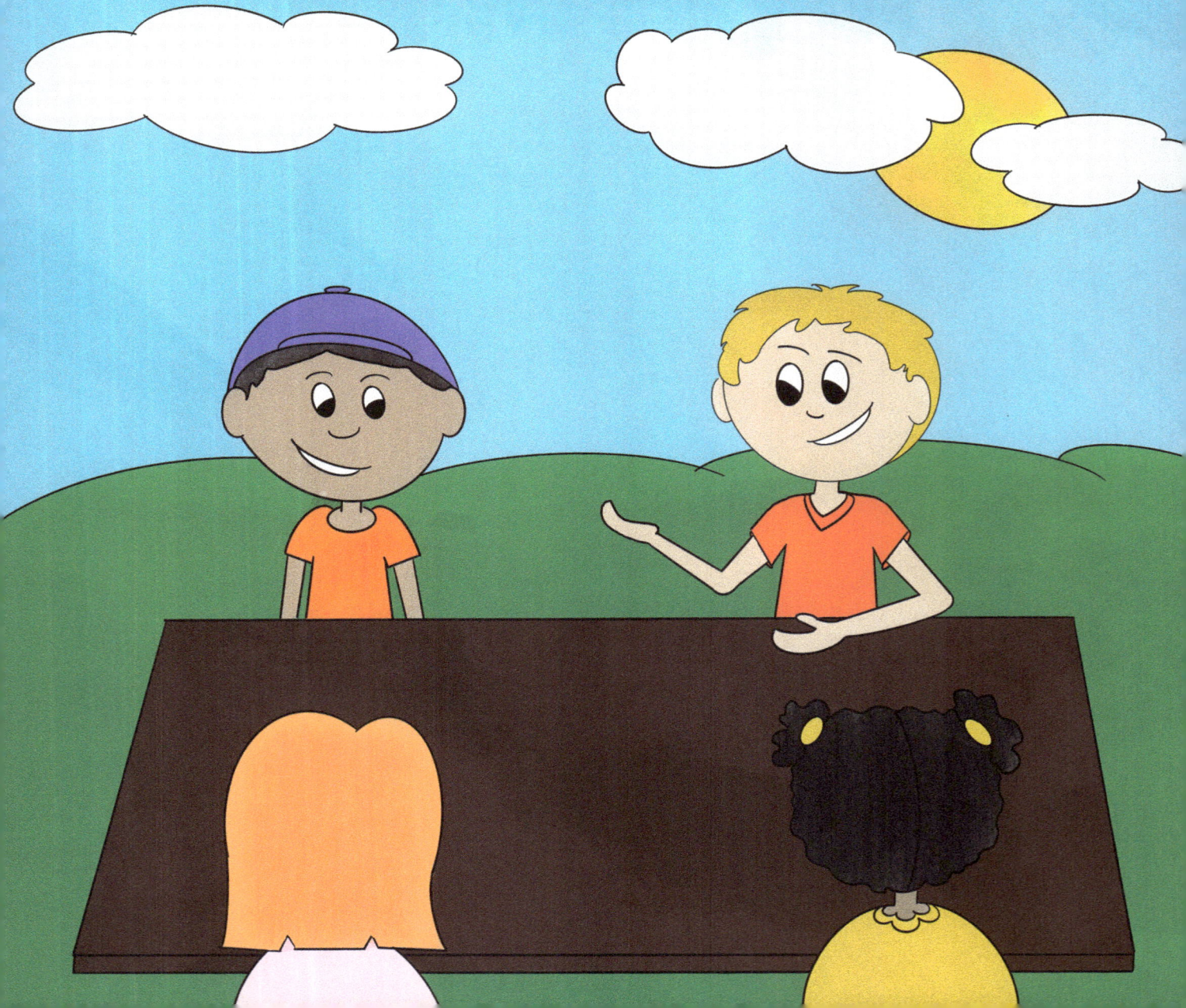

It helps us relieve stress. Constant stress can make us and our lil' friends in our gut very sick, which makes us sick."

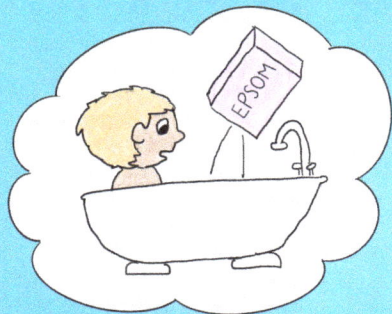

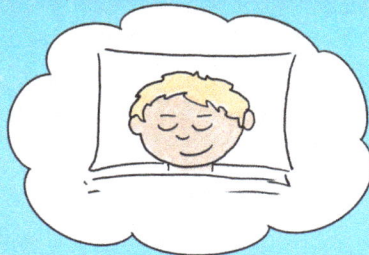

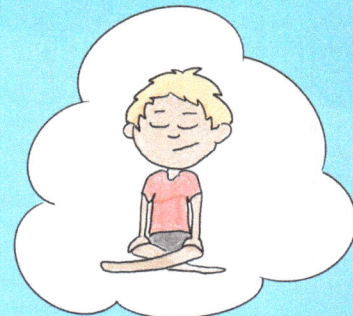

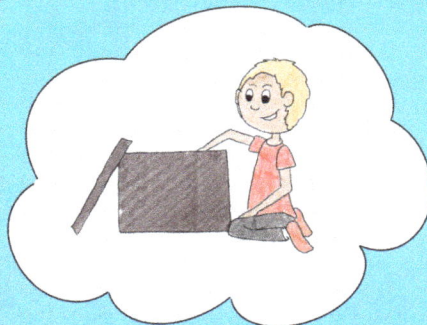

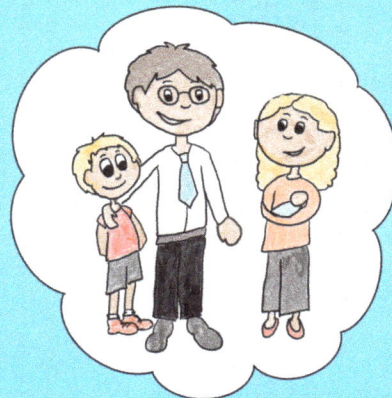

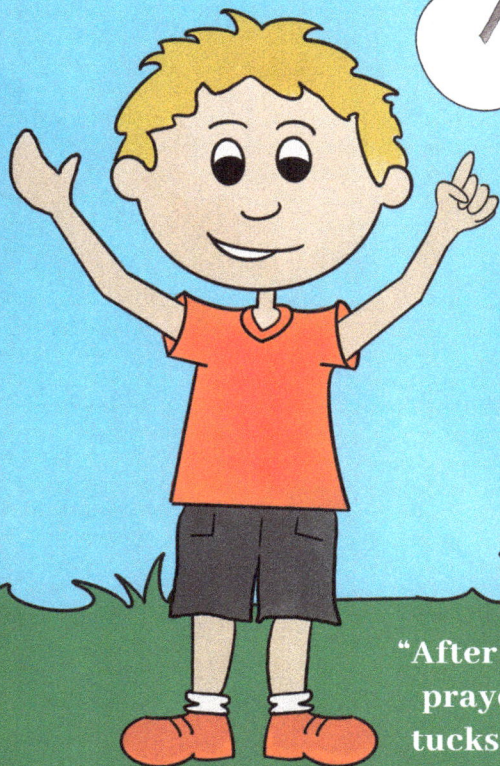

"After that, we go take a bath with Epsom salt. I love my baths! They are really healing and can help me sleep better."

"After my bath, my mom reads a bedtime story, we say a prayer, thinking about all our blessings, and then she tucks me in." Sleep is really important because it helps us grow and stay healthy in every way.

Adam was so impressed his friends knew so much about taking care
of their bodies. He loved his body as well.
"That's so easy, then why do we get sick?"

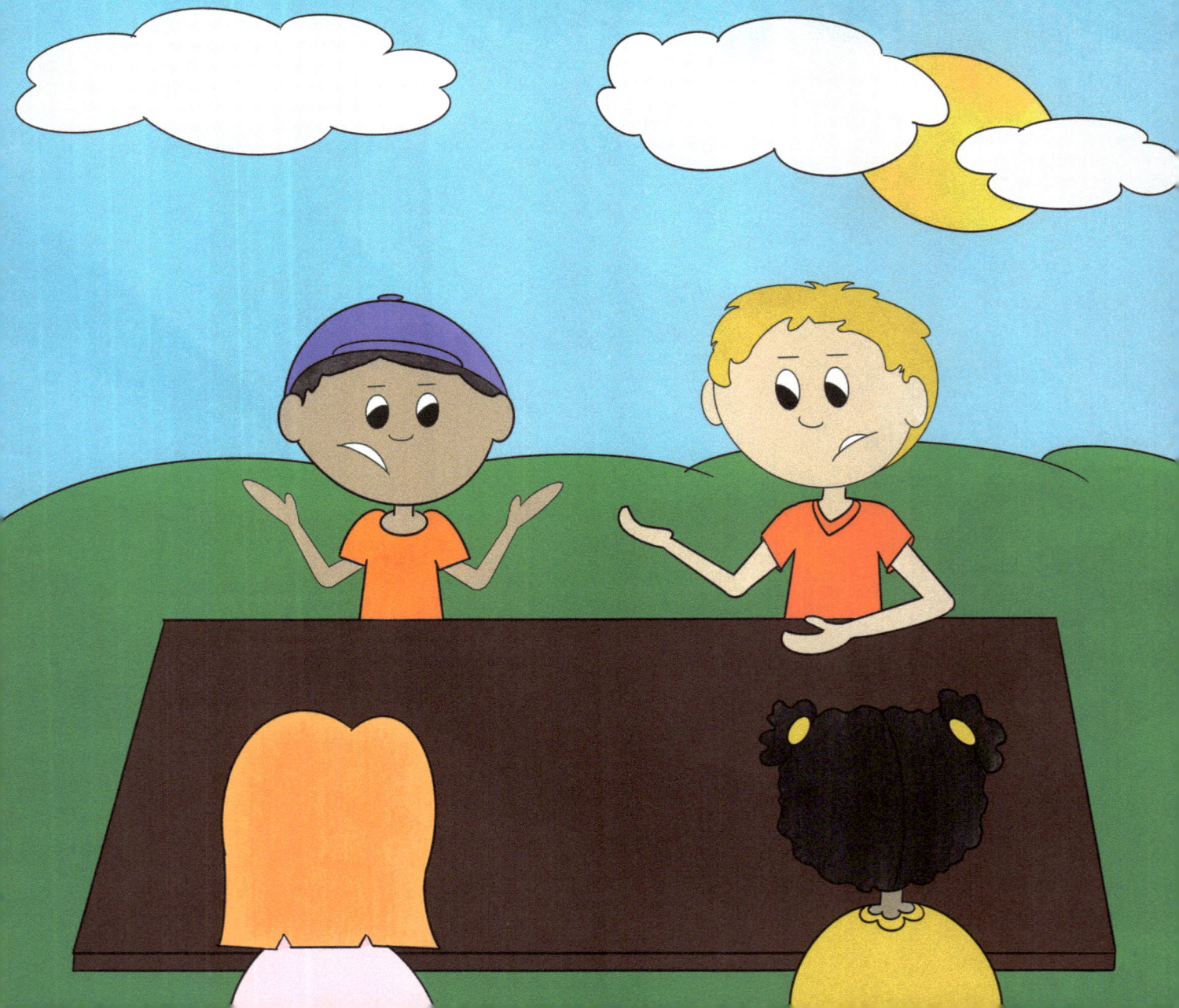

Noah tells the group, "my doctor says we can get sick if we have

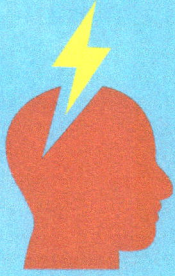

too much stress.

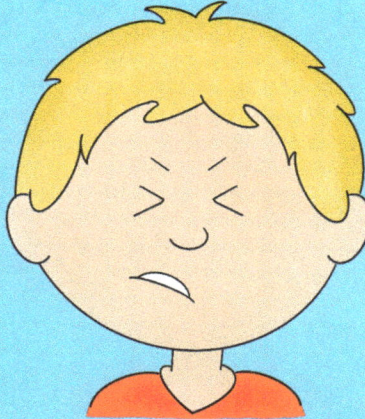

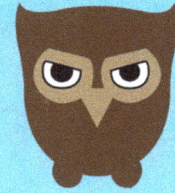

don't eat enough veggies, proteins, and healthy fats,

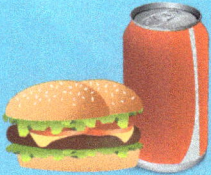

don't sleep,

have bad food,

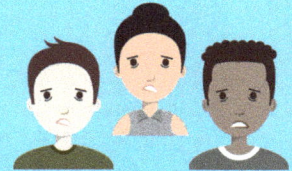

have mean friends,

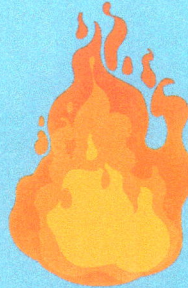

our gut gets sick,

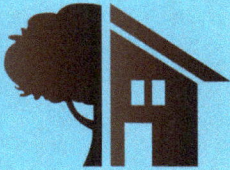

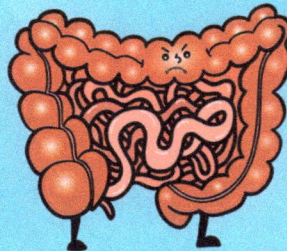

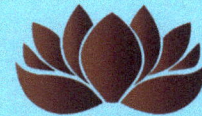

exposed to toxic chemicals,

or are not thankful.

That then starts the bad fire in the body, which can cause tummy aches, headaches, ear infections, rashes, allergies, constipation, tired or getting sick all the time and so much more. We just have to listen to our body."

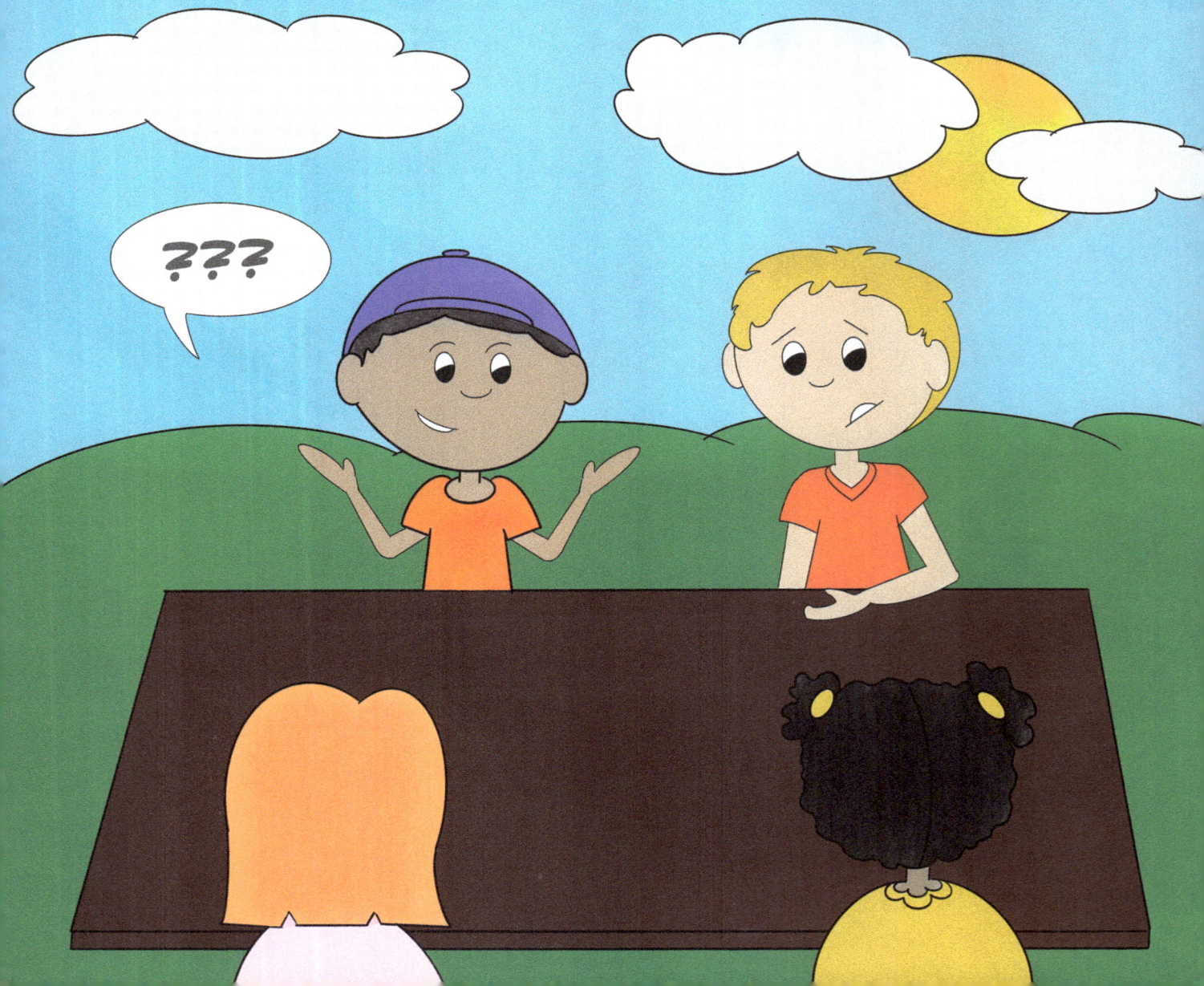

Food can either keep you healthy or make you sick.
I watch to see how the food affects my body, and if I don't feel good after eating it, I don't eat it anymore.

Foods that are genetically modified, foods with chemicals and foods with gluten/grains, dairy and sugar can make my friends sicker."
Adam made a face of disgust. "These foods have been so changed and are toxic. Ewww! I don't want to eat toxic artificial food and food that has been changed."

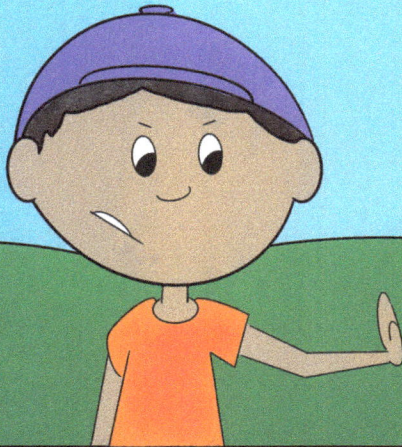
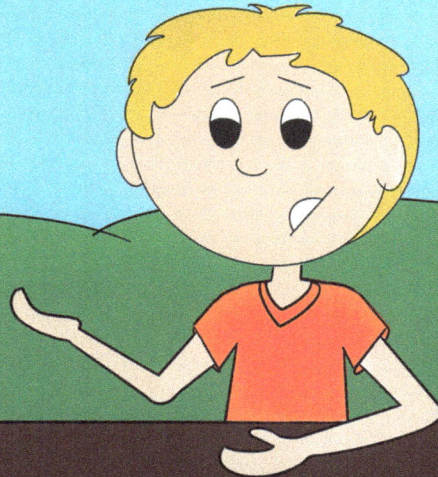
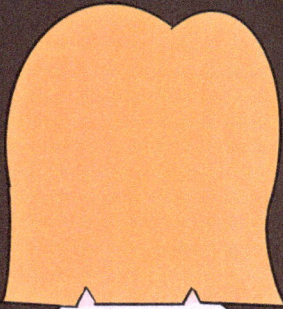
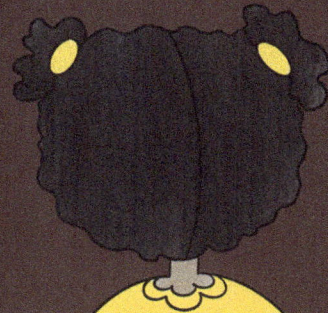

"Everyone is different, but if we take these foods out, and focus on putting my body back into balance, we can start to put out the fire in the body and feel better again.

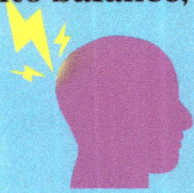

STRESS MANAGEMENT

HAPPY GUT

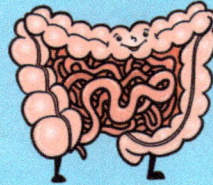

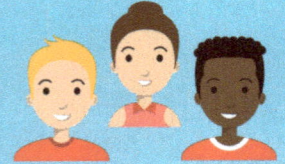

PLAY WITH GOOD FRIENDS

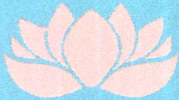

GRATITUDE

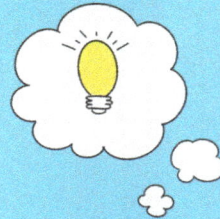

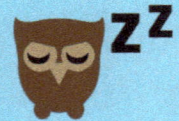

SLEEP

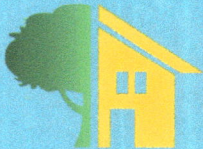

CLEAN ENVIRONMENT

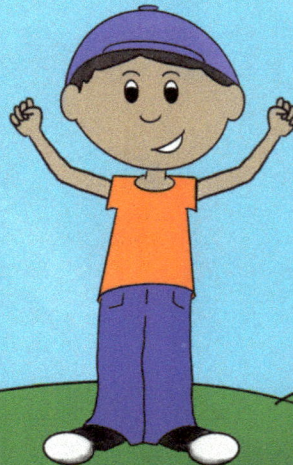

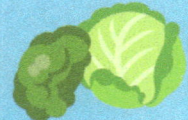

REAL FOOD & DRINK

I make sure I eat real pure food, drink lots of bone broth, meditate, play with good friends, be thankful, stay away from chemicals, and sleep well. I also take my vitamins, to fix what my body doesn't have enough of, but needs to heal, like probiotics, vitamin D, and fish oil. So easy! That is what I did, and now no more rashes or anything!"

Adam was so excited to learn so much from his friends.
He was going to start today!
At the picnic, he focused on all the things he was thankful for. He ate lots of
veggies, clean protein, healthy fat and some colorful fruit for his lunch.

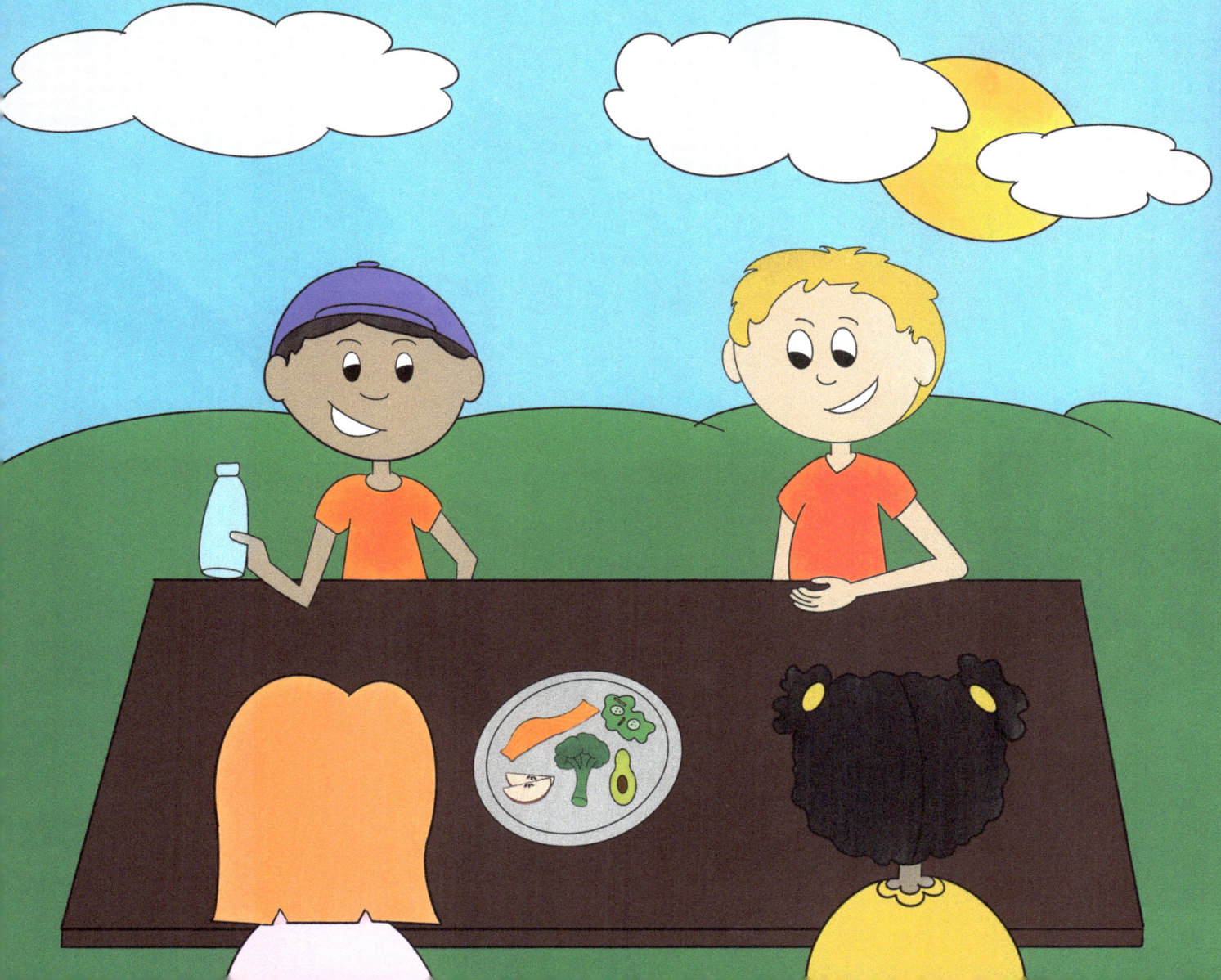

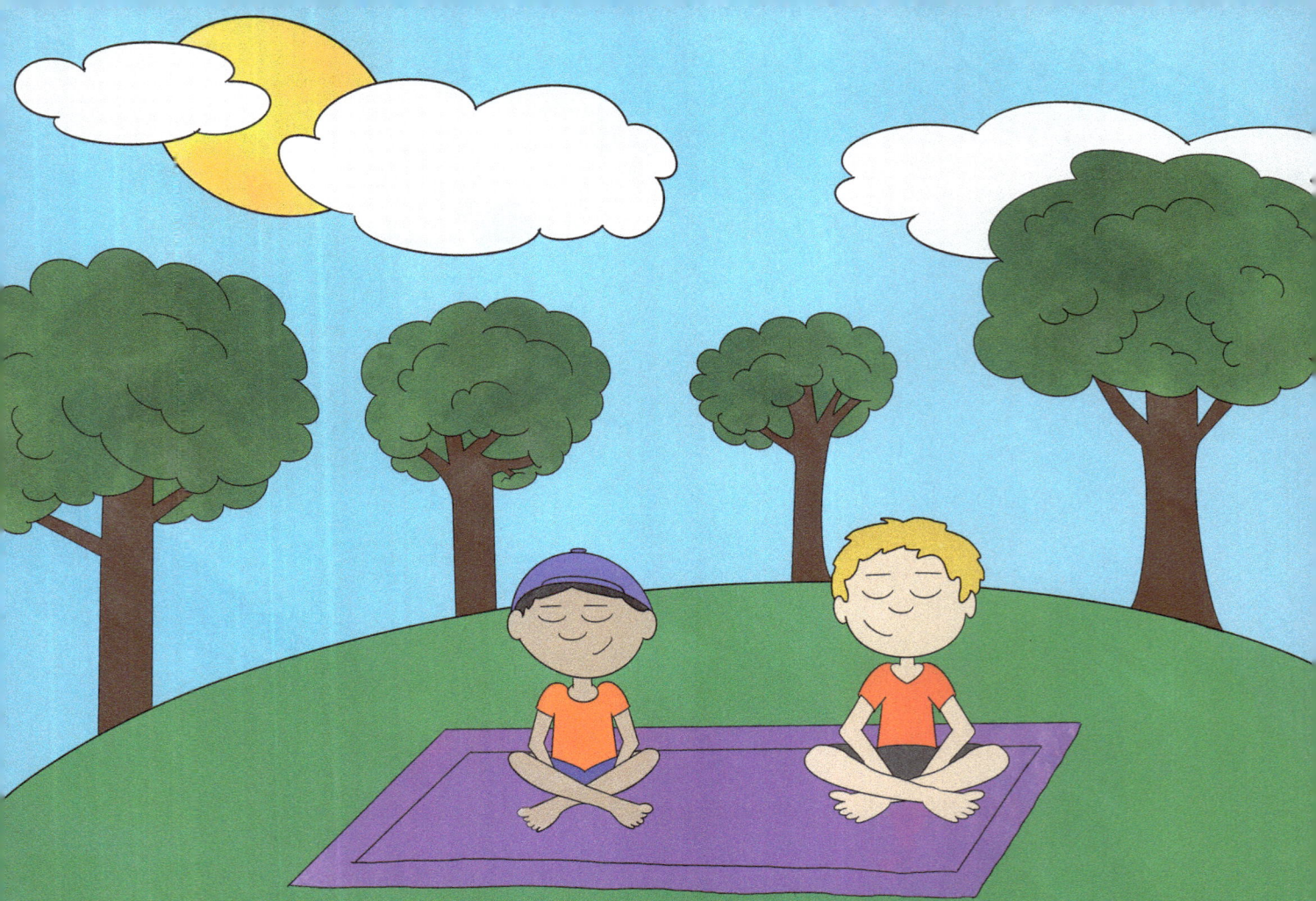

Adam also walked around outside without his shoes
and Noah even started to teach him how to meditate.

After the picnic, Adam taught his mom everything he learned. She was so surprised that these children even taught her so much! Adam's mom took him to Noah's holistic medical doctor and after some time, his symptoms started to get better. Adam was so excited that something so simple could be so effective.

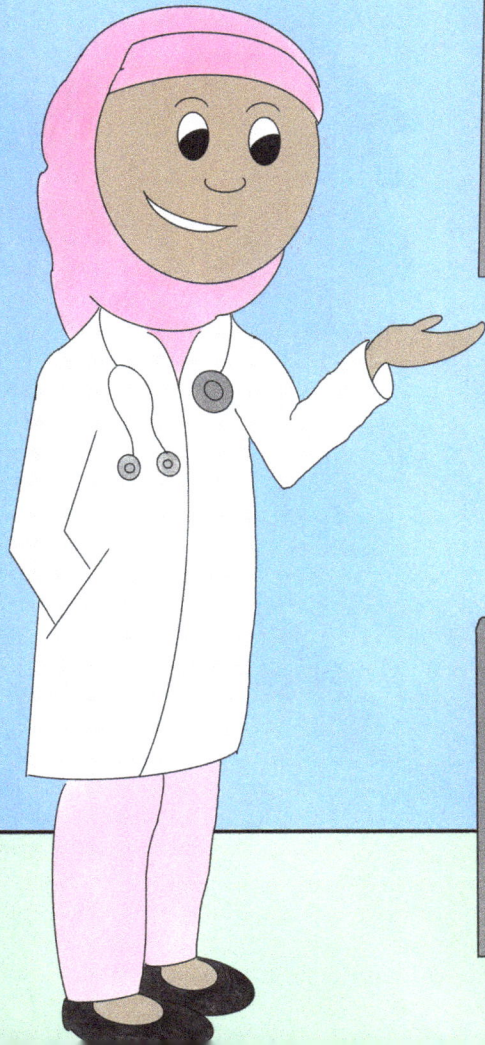

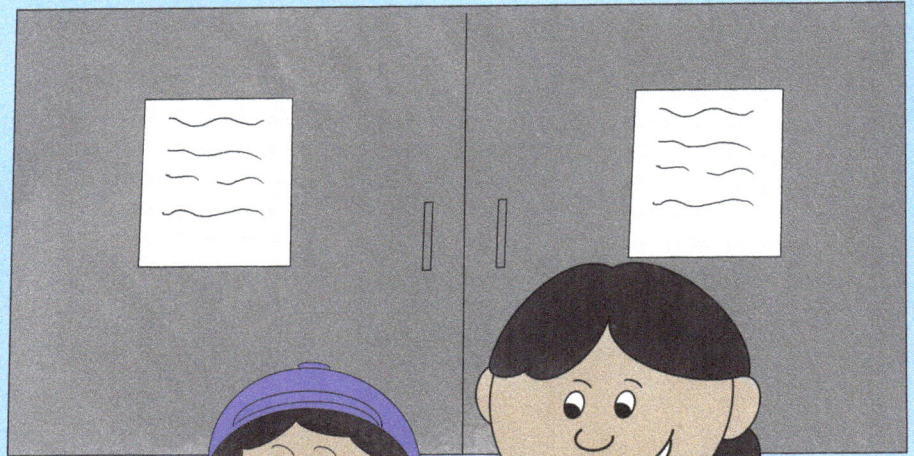

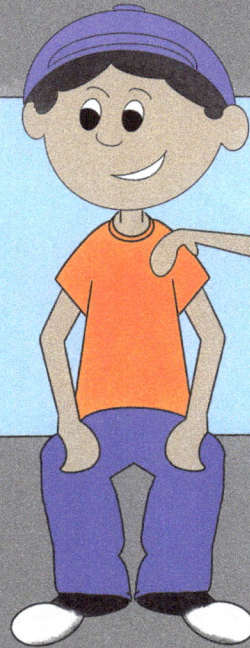

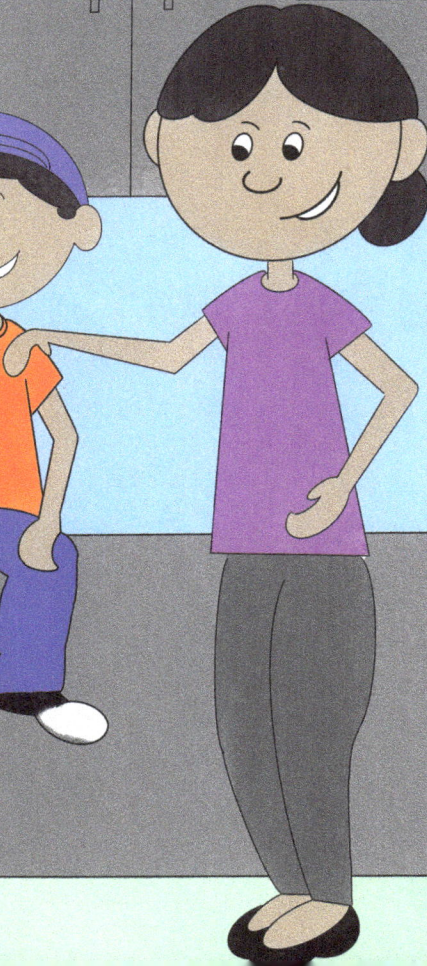

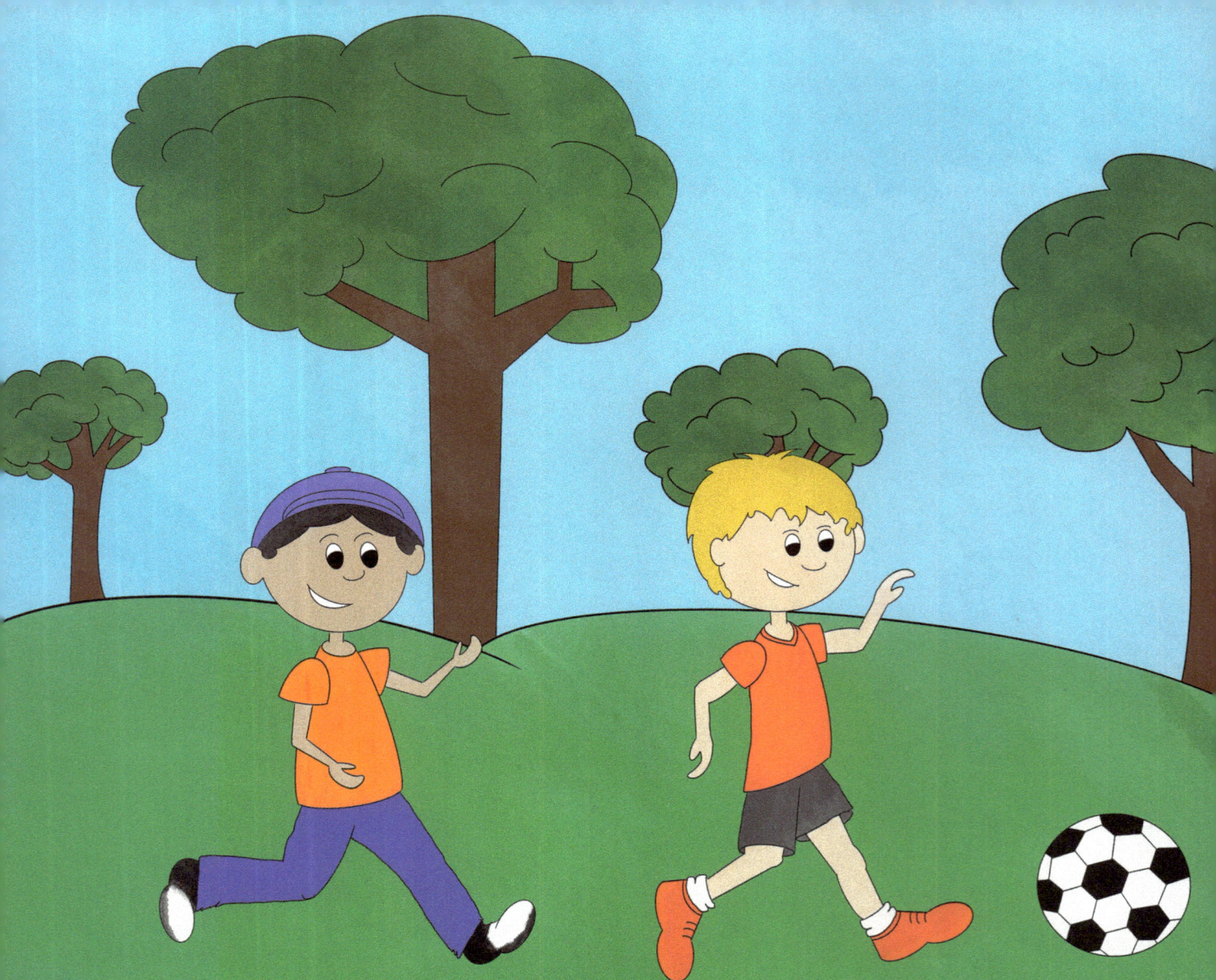

Adam's energy, rash, allergies and breathing issues continued to improve!
Adam learned to listen to his body.

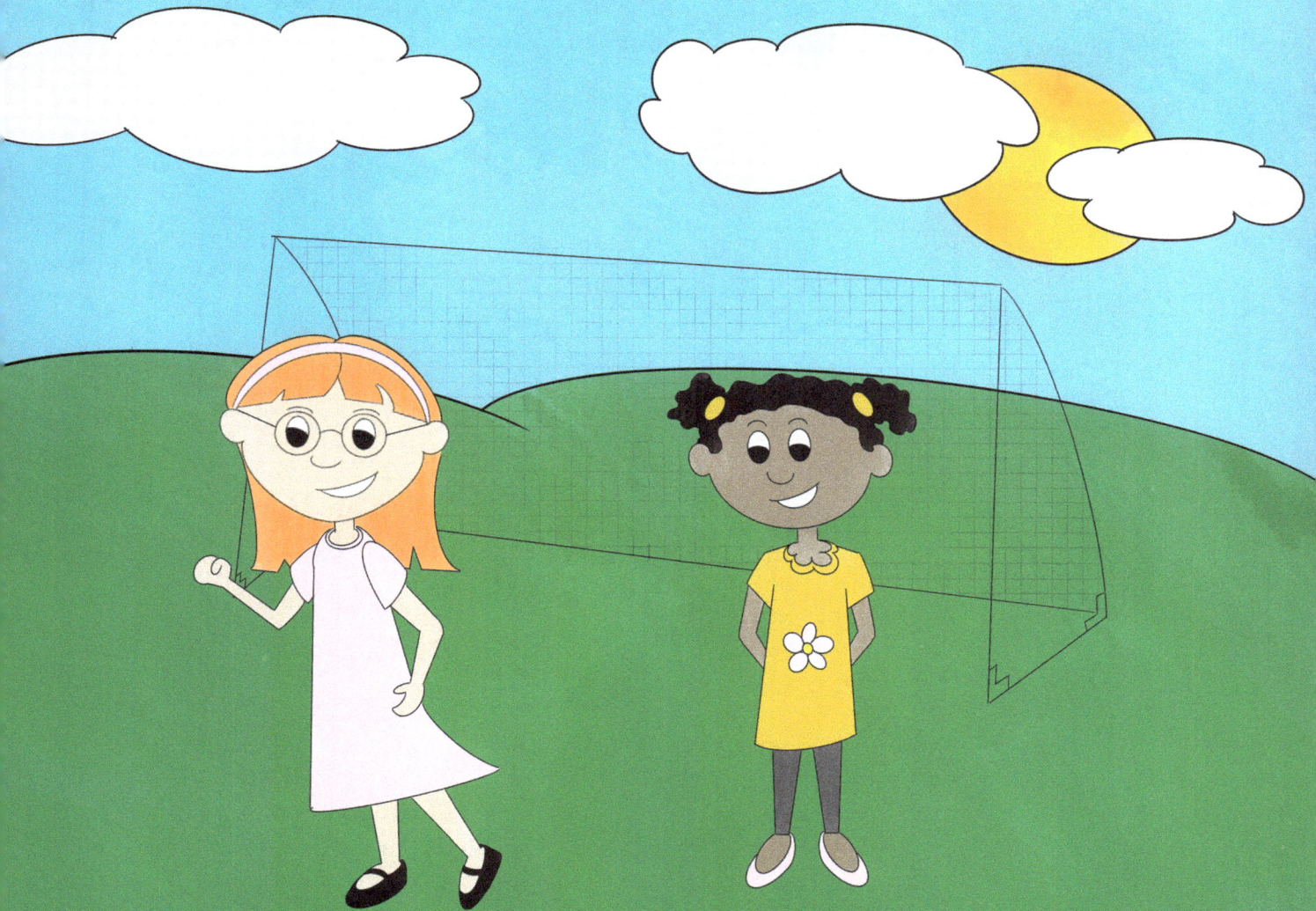

He finally felt like he was back in charge of his own health.
It was so easy to be healthy!

"I don't want to get sick. Our health is a blessing and a gift that not everyone gets. So, we have to take care of our bodies." There is so much hope!

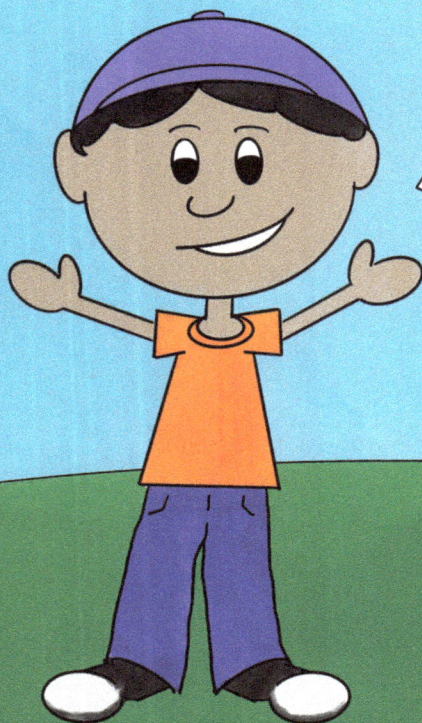

OUR HEALTH IS A BLESSING!

Adam found a new purpose, to help and educate himself and others about the power of a healthy lifestyle—Adam's Healing Adventures.

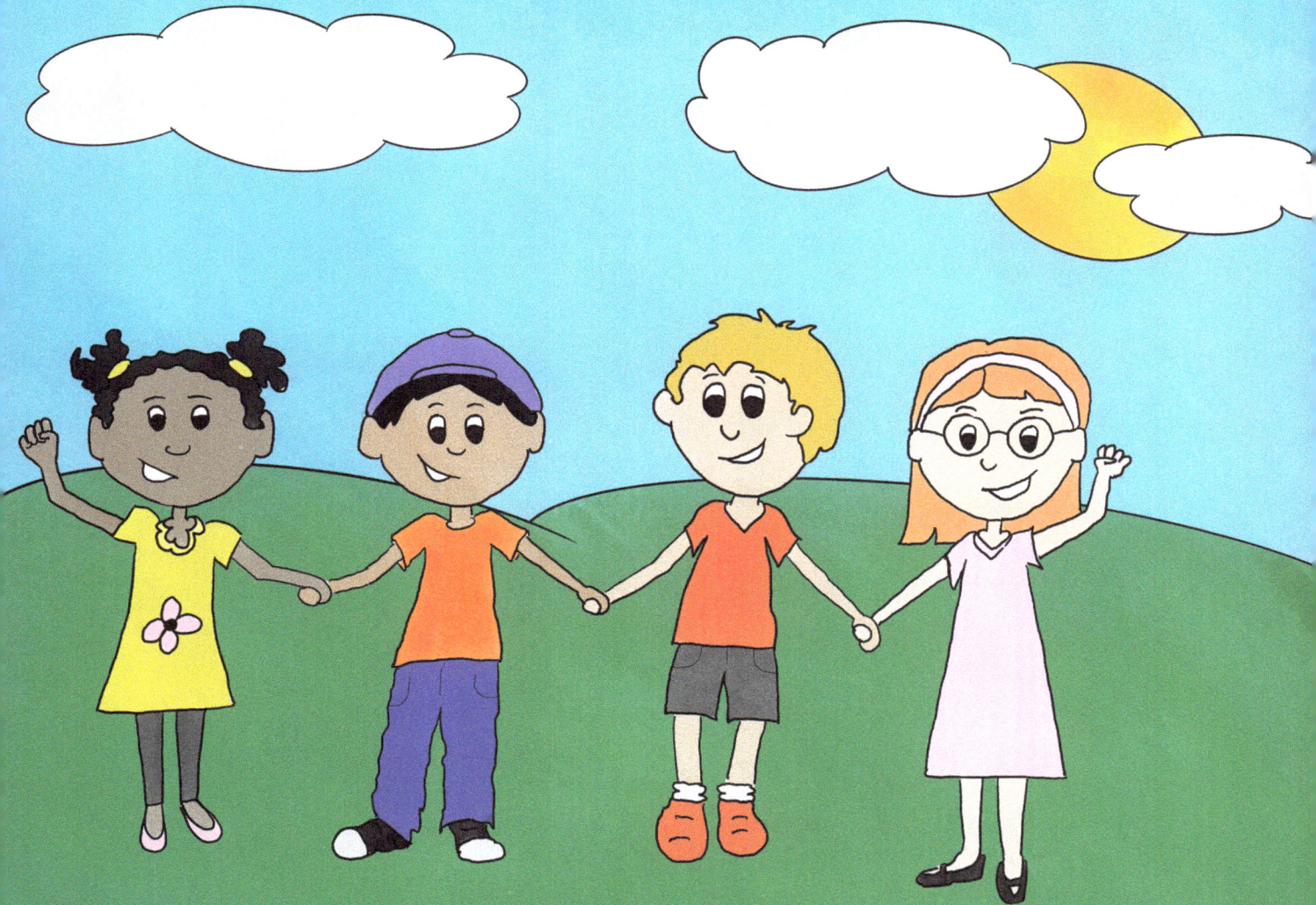

You and those around you can be that drop in the ocean of hope, creating that ripple with the potential to heal the world inside and out!

Adam's Healing Adventure Gems

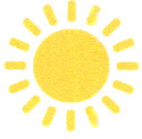

Get up each morning and say 10 things you are thankful for.

Eat the Rainbow- Focus on lots of veggies, clean protein, and healthy fats.

Drink your water.

Use all natural products around, in, and on your body.

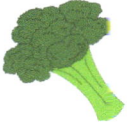

Help your body detox, with eating lots of colorful foods, Epsom salt baths and sweating daily.

Incorporate stress management techniques into your day, like prayer, mindfulness, meditation and breathing exercises.

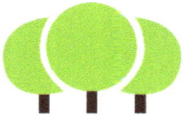

Play outdoors.

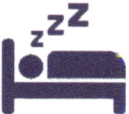

Make sure you sleep well. Sleep helps you heal.

Surround yourself with love and positivity.

THE HOLISTIC PRESCRIPTION

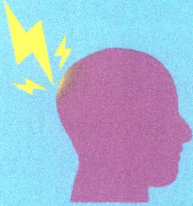

STRESS MANAGEMENT

HAPPY GUT

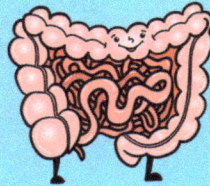

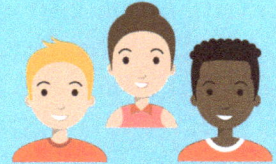

PLAY WITH GOOD FRIENDS

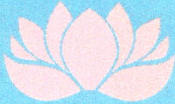

GRATITUDE

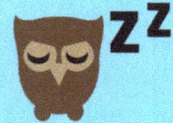

SLEEP

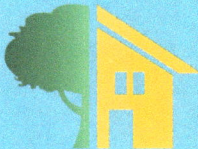

CLEAN ENVIRONMENT

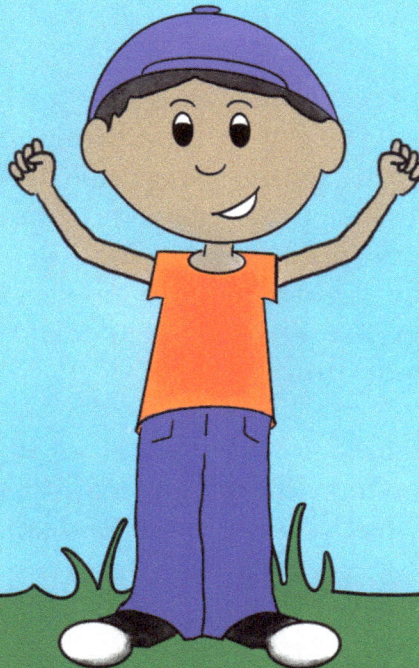

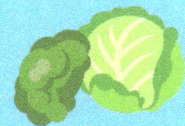

REAL FOOD & DRINK

Glossary

Inflammation: Inflammation actually means "fire inside" and it's a hot, fierce, lifesaving reaction that occurs when your body's immune system tries to fight off infections, help heal injuries and protect you from disease. There are two types of inflammation: acute and chronic. Acute inflammation (or good inflammation) lasts for a short time and serves a healthy purpose. Chronic inflammation (or bad inflammation) is a hidden, smoldering, painless fire created by your immune system as it tries to fight off modern life's daily exposures to triggers like unhealthy food, stress, toxins, allergens and an overgrowth of bad friends or microbes. Chronic inflammation drives chronic symptoms and conditions. Addressing inflammation is important to prevent, manage and/or overcome a chronic condition or symptom.

Microbiome: Human beings are actually superorganisms: we are made up of our cells plus a huge number of "bugs" or microbes that live on and inside us. These microbes (friends) are part of the microbiome. The microbiome plays an important role in our health and wellbeing.

Leaky Gut: If an imbalanced microbiome goes on for a while, it can lead to inflammation. This inflammation then damages the gut wall epithelial cells and the junctions between the cells become permeable or leaky, overtime leading to increased intestinal permeability, or leaky gut syndrome. Leaky gut syndrome is associated with a number of chronic health conditions including allergies, food sensitivities, ear infections, sinus problems, digestive issues, asthma, chronic pain, eczema and rashes, depression, anxiety, ADHD, autism, autoimmune disease and even cancer. Addressing leaky gut syndrome will help to lower overall inflammation.

Mindfulness: Mindfulness means noticing what is happening right now. It means slowing down to really notice what you are doing and what is going on in your mind, heart, and body (how you feel, what you see, taste, and smell.) When you are mindful, you are calm and focusing on the present. Mindfulness lowers worrying, stress and inflammation.

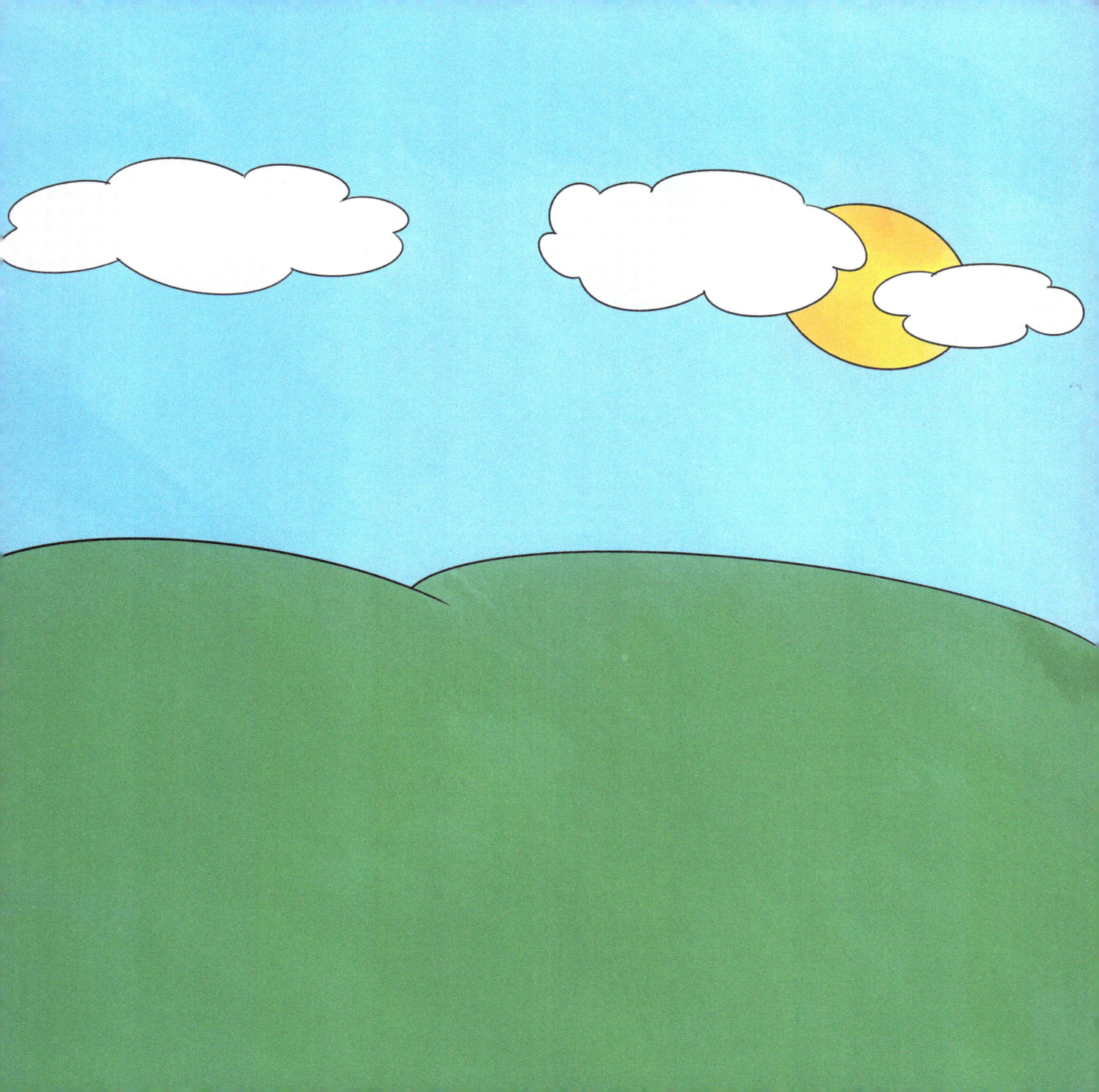

About the Author

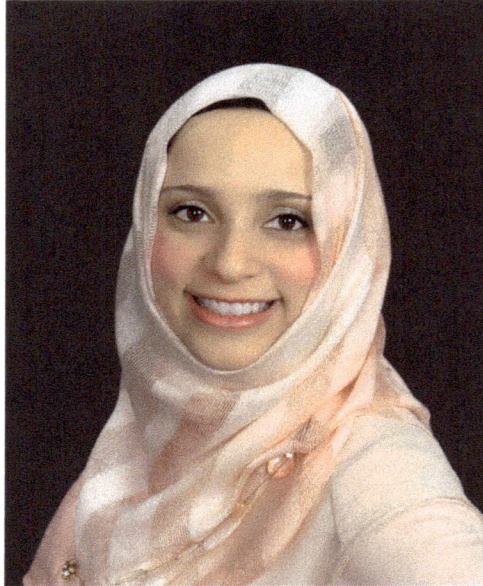

Madiha Saeed, MD, aka HolisticMom, MD, is a board certified family physician, best-selling author of *The Holistic Rx: Your Guide to Healing Chronic Inflammation and Disease*, founder of the Family Health Expo, director of education of Documenting Hope, on Wellness Mama's and Mommypotamous's medical advisory board, regularly contributes for Holistic Primary Care and has appeared on international TV, radio and print media. Dr. Saeed and her four children (Abdullah, Zain, Emaad and Qasim) speak internationally igniting the world with passion.

BLACK ROSE writing™

ISBN: 978-1-68433-524-4
PUBLISHED BY BLACK ROSE WRITING
www.blackrosewriting.com

Printed in the United States of America
Adam's Healing Adventures is printed in Abhaya Libre

www.ingramcontent.com/pod-product-compliance
Lightning Source LLC
Chambersburg PA
CBHW042350030426
42336CB00025B/3438